HEARTS

HEARTS

Of Surgeons and Transplants, Miracles and Disasters Along the Cardiac Frontier

THOMAS THOMPSON

The McCall Publishing Company

NEW YORK

Published simultaneously in Canada by
Doubleday Canada Ltd., Toronto

Library of Congress Catalog Card Number: 70-154248

ISBN 0-8415-0123-8

The McCall Publishing Company
230 Park Avenue
New York, N.Y. 10017

PRINTED IN THE UNITED STATES OF AMERICA

Design by Tere LoPrete

To my parents
and my sons

To Mom
From
Deonna

Prologue

I once knew an unimportant man who lived in a village near Kilimanjaro, where he sewed uniforms for the officers. He was a splendid tailor but he did not want to settle for that, so he spent his other hours pushing back the brush and the wait-a-minute thorns—so called because when one snared your jacket you had to stop and pull it out—searching for precious stones. When he finally found some stones one day, he fell to his knees and wept, because for the remainder of his life he would be rich and celebrated. But quickly the lions came and attacked his camp, thieves came and stole his gems, and enemies came to dispute his claims. Before a very short time had passed, his heart, as people say, broke. He died and was buried in the coffin of a tailor. I have no moral, only an observation: in the country of the unexplored, diligence can find the treasure, but only power can keep it.

I drove west, then south and down from New York. Winter gray hung stubbornly to Pennsylvania, Virginia was softening with a haze of green not quite there but in the crisp air, Georgia and Mississippi, already ripe, pink and white with first cotton. Finally Texas and its Gulf Coast, flaming with azaleas; alfalfa to the ankle, corn to the knee, new life arrogantly ahead of that not yet born in the American East.

I was driving home rather than flying because I needed to shake New York out of my head and ease into Texas. In three days on the road, one can read the signs, hear the music, see the shirt collars, accept the advice of the gas-station attendants, eat the food, drink the beer, sleep on the motel mattresses, realize once more the land of Monkey Ward and Dr. Pepper. It takes so little time to cross back to the defensive paranoia of the American South. We put it aside when we leave, but it is inbred, chronic, and almost welcome when it returns.

It is, for example, pleasant to drive in Texas not because the scenery is interesting—mostly it is not—but because the expressways, highways, roads, farm-to-market lanes are probably the best in the world (fifteen years away and one day back, and the native speaks as if he had never left). Texas has sent men to Washington—Sam Rayburn, John Nance Garner, Tom Connally, Martin Dies, and, of course, Lyndon Johnson—who patiently learned the secrets of power and patronage and, once claiming it, well served the constituents at home with surveyors, tar, and concrete.

On the spectacular straight highway to Houston, a boulevard through the forests and pine thickets of East Texas, cars shot past on this early April morning, 1970, with their windows rolled shut, drops of moisture identifying the mechanical cold within. Everything is refrigerated here because otherwise it could not exist. There is so little reason for Houston.

Because Houston had no link to the sea as most great cities do have, a canal was carved out 60 miles to the Gulf of Mexico and shippers were persuaded by charming Houston leaders to bypass the more convenient, much cheaper port of Galveston. Because the savanna land was so flat and marshy and streaked with creeks (called bayous, from neighboring Louisiana Cajun influence) that foundations seemingly could not support major skyscrapers, architects and engineers designed floating concrete slabs to anchor the tallest buildings west of Chicago. Because the air settled so heavy and humid for half the year that to be outdoors was to bathe in liquid glue, everything was air-conditioned: homes, offices, shopping centers, even the domed stadium where baseball was played: "WELCOME TO THE ASTRODOME—TEMPERATURE INSIDE, 72—TEMPERATURE OUTSIDE, 96" reads the scoreboard, and people applaud. One drive-in restaurant even offered tubes of rushing cold air, which could be stuck inside the window of that rare automobile without built-in comfort.

Because great cities must have culture, and because Houston had none to merit national attention, it was bought and paid for: first

Leopold Stokowski, then Sir John Barbirolli, finally André Previn were engaged to lead the ever-improving Houston Symphony. (Previn, it is said, was fired not because of his heavy programming of avant-garde music, nor because of his fertile alliance with Mia Farrow, but because of his guest appearance on a national television program during which he trumpeted *con brio* about his conductorship of the London Symphony, but said nothing at all—*nothing!*—about his simultaneous job with the Houstonians, who paid him more money.)

Because Houston wished to play a prominent role in the nation's burgeoning exploration of outer space, the leaders approached Lyndon Johnson, who, ever accommodating to all things Texan and particularly mindful of the suddenly undependable Democratic vote of the nation's sixth largest city, generously helped put the Manned Spacecraft Center there—ideally located some 1200 miles from Cape Kennedy—showering hundreds of millions of dollars and datelines from the cosmos, making it, of all things, Space City.

The comparison is made between Houston and Los Angeles because of the urban sprawl—Houston has 486 square miles within its city limits—and a rocketing population; Greater Houston, as the Chamber of Commerce likes to put it, is approaching two million people. But the comparison should not include the people themselves, because having known both cities well, I can state that there is a marked difference. The citizens of Los Angeles are hardly members of a city but participants in a condition unified by (1) the sun, when it can be seen, and (2) disasters—fires, floods, earthquakes, the terror of freeways that loop and whirl like insanely tied Christmas ribbons.

Houstonians, conversely, have a pride bordering on conceit. They are doers—and once something is done, they want to tell about it. When the city accumulated funds for a striking new concert hall, the mayor and a delegation hurried up to New York and held a breakfast press conference. I have been to cocktail parties in New York and found myself face to face with a stranger and have asked what he does and if the answer is, as it often is, "nothing," then I assume he is thinking, or is preparing to write a poem, or is extremely clever. In Houston the answer "nothing" would be greeted by a certain coldness because this restless, driving city welcomes only those who find the most oil, or construct the world's only air-conditioned dome, or manage the acquittal of more clients on trial for murder.

But none of this can explain the most extraordinary phenomenon of all: in a city where 25 years ago there was practiced medicine of the most mediocre sort—where there was but one infant medical school newly transferred from Dallas and a third-rate medical school at that; where there was no heritage of scholarly thinking, no foundation for orderly investigation; where extinguishing life by violence was far more common than investigating methods to prolong it—there sprang up in a swampy area six miles south of the heart of downtown, in fields where raccoons and water moccasins lived, a collection of medical facilities which, by 1970, had become one of the handful of distinguished medical centers in the world. At a cost of almost one quarter of a *billion* dollars, there had risen the Texas Medical Center—five large, all-purpose, general hospitals; a huge pink granite center for care of patients and research against cancer; hospitals for the eye, teeth, mind, crippled children; centers for public health, speech and hearing, rehabilitation, nursing, occupational therapy, physical therapy, the biomedical sciences and, dominating all—the heart.

In less time than it takes to age a good bottle of wine, Houston found itself with not only *the* most celebrated, but the *two* most celebrated heart institutes extant, standing side by side, headed by two master surgeons, Dr. Michael Ellis DeBakey and Dr. Denton Arthur Cooley, who for years had worked across the same operating table, who had become estranged, who had become pitted against each other in a passionate and poignant encounter, and who now loathed each other so that they did not even speak.

In the medical history of the city, DeBakey had come first, lured to exploding Houston in the boom years of post-World War II, brought from his native Louisiana by a consortium of doctors and civic leaders who required a force to weld a department of surgery for the infant Baylor College of Medicine. A quarter of a century ago, surgery was not the glamorous specialty it is today. Surgery was performed chiefly by general practitioners and the notion of training medical students to do nothing but cut and sew was not widely accepted.

DeBakey immediately stumbled into hostile walls, partly because of his passion for the surgeon's art and the position he felt destined to secure for it—and himself—in the course of medicine, partly because of the manner in which he sought it. At one hospital where he began operating, DeBakey observed some of the other surgeons at work and told them bluntly that they were butchers who operated when it was not necessary. At another, the staff doctors soon grew so angry with the slight, dark, hard little man that they sought to oust him. He was, they said, a tyrant: he had too many patients, he dominated the schedule, the nurses disliked him, he was disrupting the silent sanctuary that medicine was supposed to be. Moreover, they did not say it, but they considered him, the son of a Lebanese immigrant merchant, to be an outsider. He was not a regular Texan. He was intruding on them. The chief of surgery at the hospital listened quietly to their complaints and finally rose. "Mike DeBakey," he said, "may well be everything you say he is. But he may also be possessed of greatness. He may contribute something historic to medicine. Let's pull in our horns and tolerate him."

In the decade that followed, DeBakey built a department of surgery at Baylor and at the Methodist Hospital, which was to become one of the most celebrated in the world, a galaxy of young stars that revolved around the blazing sun of the brooding, exasperating man from Louisiana. DeBakey chose as his specialty occlusive disease, the building up of deposits in the bloodstream that lead to strokes or heart attacks or gangrene and amputation. He propounded his philosophy, which was to change the course of medicine: "Occlusive disease is segmental; it does not occur all over the body at the same time. You don't have to know the cause or the prevention. You bypass it, literally."

In the 1950s, Houston became the world capital for bypass surgery. DeBakey and his men devised grafts, first from the flesh of dead men, later from plastics, to sew into a threatened body and send blood detouring around an obstacle. In the mid-1950s, a remarkable device called a heart-lung oxygenating machine—known in the heart world as simply "the pump"—was developed elsewhere but so perfected in Houston that for the first time in the history of man, the surgeon was able to stop the heart and enter its quiet depths to repair the holes or deteriorating valves or redirect the flow of blood.

The doctor who became the world leader of surgery within the open heart was not Mike DeBakey, but a young disciple, Denton Cooley, who had been born in Houston to a family of wealth and social prestige. While DeBakey continued his pioneering work on the vessels of the body, Cooley plunged into hearts. Hundreds of cases became thousands, and in a city where to be first was cherished, nothing could compare with the inventory of human hearts that Cooley had repaired.

The older man, it was said, first encouraged, then was proud of, but finally became jealous of the work of his protégé—and of the man himself. Cooley was very much a Texan, very much of the regular order, very much favored by society and by nature which had blessed him with tall, powerful beauty.

The younger man broke with DeBakey in the early 1960s and moved his practice to neighboring St. Luke's Episcopal Hospital of Houston, only a hundred yards or so away. DeBakey rapidly turned *his* attention to heart surgery and quickly became as acclaimed as the youth who had left him. The years would bring them their own individual great houses of surgery, conceived and dedicated to healing the human heart and diseases of the vessels that serve it, but the years would bring as well a feud unprecedented in science, a feud more angry, more poignant, more useless than Freud's sorrowful estrangement from his disciple Jung.

In the words of one Houston physician who had observed De-Bakey and Cooley for years, "You see, Denton not only stole Mike's heart, he broke it."

PART ONE

CHAPTER

1

On Easter afternoon, 1970, in the paneled chapel of St. Luke's Episcopal Hospital in Houston, a brief and moving memorial service was held for Leo Boyd, a once strapping Canadian railroad man who had lived for sixteen mostly anguished months with the heart of an illiterate Mexican peasant woman within his chest. In his last moments, Boyd was comatose and he began to twist and turn. His wife, Ilene, reached as she had so many times before for the Panic Button beside his bed, but her sister's arms held her back and this time Boyd opened his eyes, shut them, and died. He had been Dr. Denton Cooley's longest surviving transplant and he was the last of twenty-one men, women, and children to die.

The next morning, in neighboring Methodist Hospital—more particularly in its adjoining wing called the Fondren-Brown Cardiovascular Center, a $20 million house of science and surgery created by Dr. Michael DeBakey—there came a telephone call that caused grave concern to *his* transplant team. They had transplanted only twelve hearts, but two of their patients were still alive some eighteen months postoperatively and both had long since returned to their homes and were leading fairly normal lives. Dr. Ted Diethrich, one of DeBakey's aggressive junior surgeons, took the call, which was from Phoenix, and when he hung up, his tanned, boyish face was twisted into annoyance and exasperation. He walked into the bullpen, an outer office where x-rays are studied and where young doctors and students sit for gossip and coffee.

"I just heard that Bill Carroll read about Leo Boyd's death and got despondent," said Diethrich. "Apparently he went out bar-hopping and in about the fourth place passed out. They thought he was just another drunk and God knows how long it took them to learn he was a transplant and get him to the right hospital."

"You going up there, Dr. Diethrich?" asked Jerry Naifeh, a second-year medical student who had been infatuated with surgery even before he entered medical school. He had spent one summer in Cooley's operating suites holding the sucking machine, a hose that withdraws excess blood from the chest cavity to keep the field clean for the surgeon.

"I can't," said Diethrich. "I've got too many operations here. I'll have to stay in touch on the phone." Diethrich had been a principal planner of DeBakey's transplant program and had actually put the new heart into Carroll's body and nursed him through the rejection periods. "Damn," he said morosely as he left the bullpen. "Damn. Damn. Damn!"

There were eight or ten people in the bullpen and they were waiting now for DeBakey to come out of his office for the precise ritual known as afternoon patient rounds. There was a new resident from Arkansas and today was his first chance at guiding the Professor, as DeBakey is known, up, down, and around the stairways, corridors and mazes of the three buildings over which his patients were scattered. DeBakey uses the giant Methodist Hospital, its adjoining Fondren-Brown wing, which is a self-contained hospital, and the Methodist Annex one mile south, a former nursing home taken over and refurbished to house patients during the diagnostic, preoperative period.

One of the things DeBakey pioneered is volume surgery. In the mid-1950s, the Mayo Clinic became renowned for large numbers of operations, but only those procedures—gall bladders, lung removals, and so on—that other surgeons were doing. DeBakey's volume, which stunned the medical world, was aneurysms and vessel work, then the most sophisticated and daring of operations. DeBakey did as many cases in one month as some surgeons did in a year.

The new resident, Dr. Jerry Johnson, a strong, severely barbered, raw-boned looking fellow newly back from Vietnam, was silently going over his list of patients and praying that he knew any detail DeBakey might ask about one of them. There was a rumor among the staff that DeBakey might be leaving this week on a long European tour. The staff looked forward to long absences because it cut down the patient load. Unfortunately for them, however, DeBakey did not announce his frequent departures for guest lectures, honors acceptances, and fund-raising appearances. A few years ago there had been large three-months-at-a-glance desk calendars on which De-Bakey's commitments were entered. Two were on desks outside his office and they were among the most heavily read documents in the hospital. But one afternoon he came out and gathered them up and since then has kept his schedule to himself.

Sylvia Farrell came into the bullpen looking cheerful with a new bouffant hairdo. She poured herself a cup of black coffee, put her hands on her hips and quickly appraised the preparations for the Professor. Once she had been a floor nursing supervisor but now she had responsibilities for everything from driving DeBakey to the airport to booking hotel rooms for patients' families to acting as mother hen to the younger doctors. She was a plump, effusive woman who could read, sometimes even predict, her boss's moods better than anyone else. To Dr. Johnson she said, "He'll probably only want to see the post-ops tonight, but you'd better have the other x-rays ready just in case."

Johnson nodded and hurriedly began arranging a large stack of x-rays in their manila folders. By the time they got to DeBakey, many patients had been in and out of hospitals for years and their accumulated x-rays were as thick as a family album. Sometimes DeBakey would only want to see that very morning's x-rays, sometimes he would want to observe the course of a disease by looking at x-rays for the past decade. The resident had to have them available—and available instantly—whatever.

A half dozen conversations, including some pleasant kidding of Diethrich's stunning Peruvian secretary Marguerita, because she had landed a medical student and would shortly marry him, expired in mid-sentence. DeBakey's door, 30 feet away, had opened. DeBakey came out, turned around and locked his door with a set of keys attached to his belt—he enters and leaves his office 30 times a day and never fails to lock it after him—and came wordlessly into the bullpen. He sat down and his staff gathered formally behind him. Johnson placed a neatly typed list of patients before him. These made up the patient census—everybody DeBakey has in the hospital—with a few lines after each name detailing disease, progress, treatment. There were also one or two names with nothing but a cryptic "HELLO" typed in capital letters following them, indicating to DeBakey that these are prominent patients, not necessarily *his* patients, but ones he might wish to stop in on for a goodwill appearance.

DeBakey asked a few questions that Johnson answered well—patient histories, how they appeared when they entered the hospital, whether an arteriogram—in which dye is inserted into a vessel and x-ray pictures taken—had been done. He frowned but said nothing when Johnson slapped an x-ray onto the viewing screen backward, and then stood up and quickly rushed from the room. The delegation fell in after him by rank, first Sylvia, then Johnson, then eleven other staff doctors and two visiting physicians.

DeBakey always walks tilted slightly forward with his head bent as if encountering a north wind. One would never expect him to run into anyone because his approach is made known by the circles of power which dance visibly about him. He is a slight, short man with a body of steel, a face dominated by a hawk nose that presumably marks his Lebanese ancestry but that fits more the Indian-head nickel. The photographer Karsh likened the profile to an Assyrian frieze from Nimrud in the British Museum, but eyes cannot be carved in stone and DeBakey's eyes are commanding, magnified out of proportion behind thick trifocals. I have always worried about men with eyes larger than mine because I assume they can see more.

On this spring day, DeBakey was wearing his scrub suit with his white lab coat thrown over it, the initials M.E.D. embroidered in black at the pocket. M.E.D. was everywhere—on strips of tape at the foot of patients' beds, on charts, on doors—initials dominating this empire as SPQR did ancient Rome.

Refusing to wait for an elevator, DeBakey threw open a stairwell door and bolted up, two or three steps at a time. There are those not impressed by DeBakey who suggest he bolts faster when the press or a VIP is around, but I disagree. He always bolts, he cries, he seizes, he whirls; verbs of passivity rarely describe him or his movements.

In the Intensive Care Unit on the surgical floor, he checked a dozen patients recuperating from surgery. At one bed he asked a man wearing an oxygen mask to squeeze his hand, and the man did so firmly. DeBakey's face softened into a smile. At the next bed he bent down and shouted the patient's name and the man responded in a fuzzy voice. Heart-surgery patients normally stay in the Intensive Care Unit about 48 hours, until they are completely awake from anesthesia and extubated, able to breathe without the respirator, which has worked for them since the commencement of the operation.

Everyone seemed to be progressing well except Signor Montini, a youthful Italian who had arrived in Houston in massive heart failure from two deteriorating valves in his heart. Impassively DeBakey listened to the heart into which he had replaced the mitral and the aortic valves that morning, then he knelt down and with a hint of annoyance saw that the urine bottle beside the bed was almost empty with scant fluid in the drainage tube. Passage of urine is a vital sign after heart surgery, indicating that the kidney is functioning well and receiving a good supply of blood from the reconstructed heart. It was obvious that this heart had not yet adjusted to its new hemo-dynamic system.

Montini was in his early thirties with a thick shock of dark curly hair. He was semiconscious, and now and then he would, with great effort, raise his right hand and look with wonder at the fingernails. "They've been blue so long that he can't get over the fact that they're pink now. They're getting blood after the operation," said Dr. Reed, the resident spending an unbroken 30-day-and-night tour of duty in Intensive Care Unit as part of his three months on the DeBakey service.

Now word was spreading through Fondren-Brown, into adjoining Methodist, and through the Methodist Annex a mile away, that De-Bakey was making rounds. Nurses hurried down corridors shutting the doors of patients who were *not* on DeBakey's service so they would not come into the halls and stop him for autographs. In the annex, a loudspeaker intoned, "Will all of Dr. DeBakey's patients quickly and quietly—and immediately—go to their rooms."

When he was done in the Intensive Care Unit, DeBakey stopped briefly in a nearby room to talk to his wife, a handsome and gentle Southern lady who had that day checked into the hospital with a minor complaint. "Perhaps she wanted a chance to see her husband," a nurse suggested quietly, mindful of the normal eighteen hours a day, seven days a week DeBakey lives in his hospital. Mrs. DeBakey had been known to attend teas and draw wives of young doctors into corners and tell them, in effect, "There's still time; don't let your husband become so committed to his job that you never see him." There are four DeBakey sons and they have not been able to claim a proportionate amount of their father's time. None has chosen a career in medicine.

The rounds stretched on. DeBakey made an unexpected stop at the room of Howard Stapler, whom he introduced as "a brave soldier, a very brave soldier."

"How is that, Dr. DeBakey?" I asked.

"This brave soldier is waiting for a heart transplant."

Stapler nodded his head and reached out to take DeBakey's hand. He was a man old beyond his years; he looked 65, he was not yet 50. He had sagging wrinkled skin that made his face seem to be melting wax and there were uneven tufts of stone-gray hair. Much of it had fallen out in adverse reaction to drugs. He was from a small town in Indiana, and he had been in and out of hospitals with his deteriorating heart for almost a decade. He had read so much literature on his condition that he had become efficient with cardiac terminology, almost like a prisoner who becomes a jailhouse lawyer writing habeas corpus petitions to the court.

Stapler was searching for a piece of paper on which he had written something he had read about a new operation. But before he could find it, DeBakey was out of the room, rushing across the second-story passageway that connected Fondren-Brown and Methodist. "When will the transplant take place?" I wanted to know.

"I don't know," DeBakey said. "Stapler's been worked up as well as anybody we have ever done, but there's no abundance of donor hearts anymore."

There was no shortage of violent death in Houston. Almost every morning the newspaper reported another murder in the city (Murdertown, U.S.A., as the local press casually refers to it), where guns could be purchased as easily as flashlights. One drive-in grocery owner that week had slain a bandit who had attempted to rob him. A few nights later, another bandit came to the same store and killed the owner.

"Yes," said DeBakey, "but they have to be killed just right before we can use their hearts."

The sixth floor of Methodist is practically DeBakey's private ward. Most patients begin their hospital stay by checking into the Methodist Annex for preliminary tests. They are then transferred to Fondren-Brown for surgery and a stay in Intensive Care. Finally they are moved to Methodist's sixth floor for Intermediate Care, followed by routine nursing in preparation for going home. The extent of DeBakey's practice could best be seen on the sixth floor. In room after room, the initials on the door were M.E.D., and in the majority of them, the atmosphere was pain tempered with exultation.

There was a battered-looking man named Templeton from a small town in mid-state New York whose leg had been saved from amputation. DeBakey had removed a portion of an artery occluded by atherosclerosis and replaced it with a Dacron graft, which restored circulation. The leg was still hideous-looking, with dead flesh flaking off and black patches of sores, and the toenails were those of a jungle animal, but he would walk on it again and the doctor in New York had wanted to chop it off. "If I could put the world on a silver platter and give it to you, Dr. DeBakey, I would," said Templeton, eyes glistening with tears.

The news was not that hopeful for Diane Perlman down the hall. There was extensive occlusion of several small blood vessels in her left leg, which made arterial reconstruction difficult. DeBakey had tried once before to build a new circulatory system in the leg, but the occlusion had returned. Once Mrs. Perlman had been a pert, slender, vivacious New Yorker who had modeled in the garment district before she married a shipper and bore two children. Now in her mid-thirties she was pale, frightened, and in pain from the red streaks which ran up and down the affected leg.

One of the horrors of atherosclerosis—the disease which affects countless millions of Americans and kills at least one million a year—

is that it not only causes heart attacks, it can treacherously shut off a blood vessel anywhere in the body and turn a leg or an arm purple-black with gangrene.

DeBakey made a gesture with his hands and the entourage backed quickly from Mrs. Perlman's room. As he shut the door and returned to sit beside her, she began to weep bitterly. DeBakey had nothing to offer but amputation. Twice this night the surgeon would return to her room and talk to her again, telling of what can be done with artificial legs, winning permission for the amputation, and cheering her to the point where she would say, "Thank God for pants suits." Her husband, a weary man in an iridescent silk suit and tinted glasses, told a nurse, "After God comes DeBakey; Diane is completely hypnotized by this man."

Jerry Johnson led the procession around a corner, paused momentarily, then pushed open a door. "This is Mrs. So and So," he said softly, giving a name uncertainly. DeBakey walked in with the name fresh on his lips and greeted a confused-looking woman who was not Mrs. So and So, but Mrs. Such and Such, and she was not even a DeBakey patient. DeBakey strode outside in anger. "You're supposed to be leading me, Doctor," he said to Jerry Johnson in a loud, withering voice that drew the attention of the nursing station, "and it looks as if I'll have to lead you instead! Now let's see if you can't do this very simple thing right!"

Sylvia Farrell interceded in a pacifying tone. "Dr. DeBakey, this is Dr. Johnson's first time," she said gently. Later she would take the new resident aside and suggest that he make a trial run every afternoon until he had the complicated routine down pat.

Every young doctor who has rotated onto DeBakey's service for the past quarter century in Houston has learned the potential traps that can be fallen into during the several miles of rounds. One new resident boldly led the procession into a new section of the hospital, became momentarily confused, then struck out confidently to what he thought was the door to a stairwell. DeBakey and half the group followed him, not into a stairwell but a broom closet, where in the half-second before DeBakey growled his displeasure, the doctor thought his heart would stop. Another now-prominent doctor remembers falling behind on rounds and trying to catch up while DeBakey flew down a staircase. The straggler lost his footing and fell,

bowling over an intern and two medical students on his way, rolling
down and down until he came to a merciful halt just at DeBakey's
feet. DeBakey stepped over him without comment and kept descend-
ing.

In mid-rounds, DeBakey went into the room of a friend, Ben Taub,
for a welcome interlude that the staff awaited. Every afternoon when
he was in town, DeBakey would stop in to visit with Taub, a multi-
millionaire patriarch near 80 who lived in the hospital in a two-room
suite with color TV, refrigerator, lounge chairs, and a courtly black
valet to attend his wishes. He was a magnificent-looking old man
with skin like rare parchment and the air of a wise rabbi about him.
His fortune sprang from importing cigars although it soon swelled
with real estate and banking, but he would prefer to poor mouth
people into thinking he was a modest tobacconist and his plain downtown office an extension of the nearby Salvation Army. DeBakey
was criticized by some doctors for permitting Taub and another
millionaire or two to live in the hospital, since none was ill with anything in particular to require constant hospitalization. But Taub and
the others had been long-time benefactors of DeBakey's projects,
indeed of all Houston medicine, and he ignored the carping.

When DeBakey first came to Houston in 1948 from New Orleans to
become chairman of Baylor's surgery department, he was dismayed
to find the school broke and without a hospital affiliation, something
as basic to medical education as a stadium is to football. Ben Taub
was a bachelor with a large personal fortune and was trustee for three
other rich estates. Moreover, he was chairman of the board of man-
agers of Jefferson Davis, at that time Houston's only charity hospital.

Within a year DeBakey had won affiliation with Jefferson Davis
for his medical school, and in the years that followed had pried
more than $2 million from Taub's purse for his projects. Taub said
he took to the brash Louisiana surgeon immediately. "He didn't care
about money," said Taub. "I know very many men who don't care
about money—and I'm not one of them because I care *very much*
about money." The two men had spent a good many early Sunday
mornings together at Taub's home before he moved into the hospital.
"Sometimes he would fly in at 2 A.M. and ring me up and I'd tell
him to come on over and maybe we could find an egg," said Taub.
"And we'd sit and talk and he would tell me about his projects and

his dreams. He's always had more things going than you could believe. I knew there would be no stopping that fellow."

DeBakey automatically took the old man's wrist to feel his pulse
and with his free hand dipped into an open box of chocolates.

Outside, Jerry Johnson was waiting slumped against a wall, his
face almost white, beads of perspiration dotting his forehead despite
the chill of the air-conditioning. One of the doctors who had been
through the ordeal tried to cheer him up. "You're doing fine," he
said. "Sometimes the old man takes a wrong turn deliberately just to
see if you're paying attention and to screw you up if you're not."
Another doctor nodded. "Just be sure not to volunteer any extra
information," he said. "I told him one night that I was concerned
about a patient's potassium level and he said, 'That's very interesting,
Doctor, now I'd like to know the potassium levels of everybody we
have in the hospital.' I ran my ass bloody all night long getting them
and the next day he never even asked to see them."

At the dead end of one corridor was a door with no name on the
outside, a giveaway that a celebrated patient dwelt inside. In this
instance it was a princess royal, the sister of the king of an obscure
Asian country—a regal woman of indefinite age whose left arm from
fingertip to shoulder was that purplish black of occlusive tragedy.
It had been treated in New York, DeBakey thought, quite poorly. He
was now prescribing drugs and waiting for the line of demarcation
to settle in, indicating the place where he would, or hopefully would
not, have to amputate. Often his cases were those that had been
botched up or ignored elsewhere and about twice an afternoon he
came out of a patient's room muttering, "Butchery, sheer butchery."

Methodist Hospital attempts to cloak famous patients—the Duke
of Windsor, Jeanette MacDonald, Curt Jurgens—with anonymity,
but DeBakey has never become exceptionally upset when their
names, coupled with his, get into the newspapers. "He is a master of
publicity," says one DeBakey watcher. "He was the first doctor to
realize what a valuable tool it could be." The two Houston papers
cover both heart hospitals as a major beat and DeBakey and Cooley's
activities produce several local stories a month. Such exposure has
traditionally outraged the Harris County Medical Society's ethics
committee, which feels the only paper a doctor's name should appear

in is a medical journal. Both men have been before the committee on publicity charges but neither pays much attention to such hearings. DeBakey usually turns the matter over to his lawyer.

A Biafran chief had been waiting all afternoon for DeBakey to enter his room and when DeBakey arrived, the splendidly muscled black man presented a new complaint. He had originally come to Houston for open-heart surgery, which was successfully over with; then he complained of a gall bladder, which was repaired; now he thought he had a hernia. It seemed he was fully prepared to stay in Methodist for years, undergoing procedure after procedure and delaying the day he would have to return to his fallen country.

The last stop was to see a woman whose mitral valve, one of four valves in the heart that control the flow of blood, needed to be replaced. The mitral, located in the heart's left ventricle, is the one most often damaged by childhood rheumatic fever. The patient was a country woman and so frightened that her huge butter-and-milk body was jerking as she listened fearfully to DeBakey's terse remarks. "We're going to fix that up for you tomorrow, deah," he said in his soft Louisiana drawl. The staff turned to one another and spoke with their eyes. This apparently meant DeBakey would not be leaving for Europe. DeBakey took her hand and patted it; she glanced down at his abnormally long, slender, almost feminine fingers, the tops heavily covered with black bristly hair. She put her other chubby hand on top of his and pressed it tightly. "Well," she said, "if that's what you have to do. . . ." DeBakey nodded. "Then," she was summoning courage and picking up speed, "you go right ahead and do it. Just make sure *you* do it. That's what I came for."

"You'll be fine, just fine," he said, almost automatically. "I'll see you tomorrow in the recovery room after the operation." The last remark was subtly important; it gave the patient a projection into the future, beyond the operation, beyond the terrible unknown of this small, tense, abrupt man who was going to cut into her heart.

On the way back to his office DeBakey suddenly said, "I'll be leaving in a few days for Europe. I'll be gone about a week. I've got to deliver a speech in Rome and then stop by Belgium to see King Leopold and Princess Lilliane. The king has not been feeling well lately." I could not tell from his routine delivery of this interesting itinerary if it was information or a boast—but he certainly looked like a court physician, scurrying off, entourage at his heels. He had seen 47 patients in 32 minutes.

In the bullpen after rounds, Jerry Johnson gulped a quick cup of coffee before setting off to make the same rounds over again, going back to the rooms of everybody DeBakey had seen and answering the questions they were too frightened to ask of DeBakey. Johnson was talking to Santiago, a handsome and intense young surgical fellow from Argentina, saying that he had decided to go into plastic surgery.

"Why?" asked Santiago, who, like most of the foreign surgeons who continually flock to Houston to hover at the elbows of DeBakey and Cooley, was totally committed to the glamour and potential of cardiovascular work.

"Because I don't want to work around really sick people. I get too involved with them." Johnson looked out the window into the parking lot. An elderly man was trying to help his wife out of a wheelchair and into his Buick. "I don't really like them. I can't get them out of my mind."

Santiago cut in quickly with his romantically accented English. "But you must leave them at the hospital when you go home at night. You go crazy otherwise."

DeBakey arrived before sunrise the next day and worked in his locked office until 7:30 when he suddenly appeared on the third floor surgical suite. He had changed from his street dress—suit custom made by a Beaumont tailor, shirt of a special light cotton made for him in New York, carefully knotted polka-dot bow tie—into his surgical scrub suit, which differed from everyone else's greens because his was powder blue, his favorite color. The blouse had a thicker layer of absorbent gauze to soak up the blood, which splatters in the best of surgeries. He was in a foul mood, which everyone sensed, probably because he was going to begin the day by amputating Diane Perlman's leg.

"I wish to God it didn't have to be done," he said, as he scrubbed in, washing the lean fingers for ten minutes, then scrubbing his nails with a throw-away plastic sponge. Up until a handful of years ago, reusable brushes and orange nail sticks were used and sterilized after every scrub, but a committee of Texas nurses had introduced the idea of disposable ones.

There are eight operating suites built in a circle around a central glass-walled control room where computers are being installed to monitor patients during their surgeries. When perfected, they will report on all the vital signs of a patient and squawk warnings in advance of a dangerous plunge in blood pressure or of an arrhythmia, the abnormal rhythm that can send the heart into fibrillation and death. DeBakey and his two junior surgeons, Ted Diethrich and George Noon, occupied four of the suites. Other members of the Baylor surgical faculty used the remaining four, turning an average of 50 percent of their fees over to the department. The eight rooms were equipped with the most magnificent of equipment, electronic innards of such sophistication that engineers had become a vital part of surgery. In mask and gown, they entered the chambers almost as frequently as the surgeons.

DeBakey pushed open the swinging doors of Room 4 and saw Mrs. Perlman on the table, already sedated and draped. Only her mottled, pink-streaked leg was exposed; the rest of her body was covered with green sterile cloths. "This is an operation of failure," said DeBakey. It took but a few minutes to cut through the flesh, and even less to chew the bone through with an electric saw. The severed leg was wrapped in a green plastic sheet and given to an orderly for delivery to pathology. DeBakey left the room and Diethrich sewed up the stump. One of the nurses was recalling another amputation, a woman who demanded that she get her leg back from pathology when the tests were completed. "That leg is still a part of me," the woman had said, "I'm going to have it buried in the family plot where I will join it some day."

At midday DeBakey disappeared. Newspapers the next day reported he gave a speech in Kansas City urging more federal money for research. He had embarked on a passionate denunciation of Richard Nixon and his budget allotments. Nixon had become the newest windmill for him to joust. And there were so many others— the American Medical Association, the local medical society, any organization or individual who differed with his strongly held belief that medicine is a right, not a privilege. He was the most towering figure in Houston medicine, but he was also the most actively disliked. A small percentage of his cases were local referrals. What affection was denied him at home, he could easily find outside its borders. A trophy case in the conference room of Frondren-Brown was filled with gold scalpels and medals and ornate scrolls attesting to his accomplishment, and the case was always lighted, like an eternal flame. "Mike DeBakey," said one of his most bitter critics, a Baylor faculty member of considerable power, "has an almost pathetic need to recrown himself every day. He will accept the invitation of some girls' school somewhere in backwoods Pennsylvania and go there and get their medal and fly home all night and charge into surgery. I cannot understand why a man of his power and prestige needs such hosannas."

In his absence, Ted Diethrich ran the service and at mid-afternoon fairly bounced out of the operating room into the coffee lounge. He had heard from Phoenix that Bill Carroll was responding well to treatment and that his transplanted heart showed no signs of damage from the bar crawl. Moreover, he had just done a surgical "first," or what he believed to be a "first."

"It was fantastic! It was the first time anybody replaced a mitral valve and at the same time cleaned out a coronary artery with gas.* I'm not sure I should talk about it until I'm sure the guy makes it. But he looks fantastic!" Ted was only 35 but looked eighteen and if he came into my room and announced he was the one assigned to remove the hangnail, I was not sure I would let him do it. But he is brilliant, already one of the recognized fast guns, and all the other fast guns have made note of him.

Signor Montini's monitoring scope, electronically measuring his heart rate, had gone all but flat. There had been no improvement in urinary output, his eye pupils settled fixed and dilated. His body had become the texture of cold sponge rubber. He was not so much a human any more as an abstract object committed to the wires and

---

* *The gasendarterectomy, or "gas" as it is called in the heart center, is a procedure developed in New York in the late 1960s. The surgeon makes an incision in a heart artery and injects whiffs of carbon dioxide gas. This loosens the cholesterol and occlusive matter and enables the surgeon to lift out the entire core thereby restoring blood flow.*

tubes and machines, which covered and wrapped his body. The ventilator that had breathed for him for almost 48 hours was still pushing oxygen impersonally into and out of his lungs, forcing his chest to rise and fall as that of a life-filled man. Dr. Reed, the resident, directed an exquisitely timed and executed attempt to resuscitate the heart. With his palms he slammed into the chest—*BAM*—*BAM*—*BAM*—at intervals of one second. A nurse handed him a hypodermic needle filled with adrenalin, which Reed plunged directly into the heart. The scope began to leap fitfully, only to settle back again. Someone else shot digitoxin to strengthen the heart into an intravenous tube; an inhalation therapist was pumping moist oxygen into the lungs.

After perhaps ten minutes, after countless scores of slams onto the chest, Reed lifted his arms, paused, looked at the scopes with puzzlement, and stopped. Nothing was said, all was lost. Within the brain —deprived now of blood for a quarter of an hour because the heart had stopped pumping it—each cell was shrinking, then turning dark as if stained blue. Each cell was shuddering and breaking up, dissolving, the nucleus disappearing into the cytoplasm, caught up in the dance of death. Millions, billions of cells, each containing DNA, the origin of life, were blinking out. Massive cell death was rushing throughout the body, extinguishing life in the kidney, then the liver, the lesser organs. Oddly, the heart, though stopped and the assassin in this murder, was one of the last to go. A remarkably hardy machine, the heart has been known to leap back into activity after arrests of up to one hour. But by then its owner would be, as Montini would have been, a vegetable; the brain can survive only four or five minutes without life-giving blood.

A nurse drew a lemon-colored curtain around the cubicle to spare other patients the sight of Montini's *bain de mort*. An orderly moved in to disconnect the machines and wires and tubes, and when that was done, he scrubbed away the medication and blood from the body. The final act was the classic drawing of the sheet across the face. The orderly pushed the bed across the Intensive Care Unit to an empty corner where a screen was placed about it. There Montini would wait until the trip downstairs to pathology—provided the family gave permission for an autopsy.

Even now there was life of a primitive sort within him. The hair follicles would continue to grow for hours, perhaps days; the nails would remain alive even longer, and his intestines would shift silently and engulf one another. Were it not for embalming fluid and the cold boxes into which the dead are put in morgues and funeral homes, growth would continue for several days.*

I watched the pageant with mute fascination. It was the first occasion I had borne witness to the actual moment of death. I had seen death before, after-the-fact death, that principal currency of journalism. I had, and I would never forget it, seen my first violent death in this very city, fifteen years ago, on my first week's work for a now defunct newspaper.

Those first dead and those dead since of traffic, riot, and war were figures in an impersonal tableau; I had no prior identification for them, and when I had come upon them, they were only to be counted and tagged and their widows telephoned for color. Signor Montini had lived! He had asked for ice in a hoarse voice, he had raised his hands to look at his nails, he had brought his heart to Houston because DeBakey could repair it, and now he was stiffening and lost.

"What did he die of, exactly?" I asked Reed.

"Pump failure," he said, but he was busy attending to a woman who was trying to climb from her bed and yank the intravenous tube from her hand.

Because DeBakey was not there, the unwanted task of telling the family fell to George Noon, one of the junior surgeons. With death the machinery of the hospital moves quickly; already the dead man's brother had been brought to a tastefully done chamber in oriental décor called the Family Room (adjacent to the Intensive Care Unit). A chaplain was beside him, as was a member of the hospital's social service staff. An interpreter was present; Methodist can summon the speakers of more than 30 languages—and has.

The moment Noon opened the door, Montini's brother could tell from his face that the day had turned dark.

"*Morto?*"

A nod.

"No!" A fist slammed into a palm.

---

* *A Baylor pathology professor was conducting an autopsy years ago when a student cried out that he felt a pulse in the cadaver. The professor hurriedly examined the "pulse" and brusquely told the student that the life he thought he felt was contained only in his own fingers.*

CHAPTER
2

Sunday was both exodus and genesis, the old patients leaving, the new ones filling their beds. Even though DeBakey had flown first to Rome, where he was to be blessed by the Pope and thence to Brussels, where he would attend a retired king, his service ebbed but slightly. In his absence, the staff admitted new patients and worked them up for DeBakey's return. Ted Diethrich and George Noon scheduled surgery as well, it being their privilege to serve both as academicians and as private doctors. In most of America's leading medical schools, the custom is for surgeons to be full-time faculty members, drawing a salary as their only income, allowing them to teach, perform operations, and remain divorced from the competitive world of private practice.

DeBakey, however, has stubbornly kept it both ways. He has never let go of his private practice, one of the largest in the world, even though he is president of Baylor Medical School and simultaneously chairman of its Department of Surgery. For more than two decades he has employed the various medical castes—students, interns, residents, and fellows, plus a full-fledged junior associate or two like

Diethrich and Noon—to assist him in running the huge census. The returns seem beneficial to all concerned: the younger men get practical experience from assisting and observing all manner of sophisticated, even avant-garde surgery; DeBakey, on the other hand, fulfills his teaching responsibilities and gets inexpensive help.

During the night a Gypsy prince—or king, his position in the tribal hierarchy seemed to vary depending upon which member of his entourage one talked to—arrived on a stretcher. He was admitted as Thomas Eglund and gave Seattle as an address. He said he had suffered a massive heart attack while on business with his tribe in Kansas and they, alarmed, chartered a plane to fly him to Houston, where he presented himself for treatment "only by the great Professor DeBakey." No one knew exactly what to do with him, so Prince Thomas was put in a room on the sixth-floor postoperative wing, a heart monitor attached to his chest. There he would wait, under observation, until DeBakey returned. A young man of only 35, the prince was obese; his blubbery body filled the single-size hospital bed and it was important that he lie still because there was no room for him to roll. He had a neat pencil-thin mustache and three rings on his left hand and two on his right, which he refused to put in his drawer.

The floor nurses spent most of the first night chasing his family out of the room. The women wore flowing, pleated skirts that fell almost to their stiletto heels; their golden looped earrings and bracelets clanked as they clattered down the quiet hallways trailing clouds of garlic and olive oil. One woman had her front teeth set with diamonds and she fairly sparkled as she begged permission to sit through the night at the bedside of her ailing kinsman.

Finally the head nurse grew weary of expelling the family. She put up a chain across the floor and threatened to notify the hospital police if they did not stop slipping down the corridors. "Your patient is a sick man and he must rest now," said a tiny Philippine nurse with a remarkably large voice. "You can visit him in the morning."

Both Methodist and St. Luke's had become meccas for prominent Gypsies. And both hospital administrations had grown wary of the tribes' boisterous cries for the best of everything—the best rooms, the best round-the-clock nurses, the most elaborate tests—and also, particularly if the outcome was unpleasant, their refusal to pay. During one Gypsy's confinement, while he was in another part of the hospital for x-rays, his relatives took turns climbing into the bed and playing with the automatic controls that made it go up and down. When a nurse demanded that the matriarch remove herself from the bed, she retorted, "We are paying for this bed, and the whole family is entitled to use it."

On another occasion, an alert member of the Methodist security force spotted one Gypsy nonchalantly pushing another in a wheelchair out the front door. Neither, as it turned out, was sick, but the chair could have been sold for several hundred dollars. Television sets, sheets, boxes of bandages, even an EKG machine have disappeared during Gypsy sicknesses. The most memorable Gypsy assault took place at St. Luke's, when one of America's major tribal kings underwent open-heart surgery. During the operation he vomited and a bit of it went to his lungs, followed by an embolism that traveled to his brain. For weeks he lay in extremis while the clans flocked to Houston. They set up tents on the hospital lawn and parking lots; one doctor left work late in the afternoon and discovered a Gypsy family feasting on roast chicken atop his Cadillac. By the time the king had reached his final hours, there were hundreds of mourning kinsmen scattered about the Medical Center, and when he finally expired, the immediate relatives refused to pay the bill because they had not received what they had come for, which was the king's successful recovery.

When Prince Thomas checked in, Methodist's Admitting Office demanded a $3,000 deposit. The family balked but came up with $1,000 in wrinkled, carefully counted out small bills and the promise to find the rest.

On a Monday morning, Ted Diethrich set into motion examinations to determine if 43-year-old Arthur Bingham, a Phoenix businessman, could be a candidate for the newest and hottest operation in heart surgery—the coronary artery bypass. This is a delicate procedure in which a vein is borrowed from a patient's leg and hooked up within the heart to give it a better supply of blood. The operation was devised by cardiologists and surgeons in Cleveland and Minneapolis, but typically the Houston heart men had begun modifying and improving and doing so many that they were becoming recognized as among the world leaders.

At its simplest, the most common acquired heart disease is narrowing of the arteries on the surface of the heart from occlusive matter—largely cholesterol. When this occlusive matter builds up to the point where it completely shuts off blood supply to a portion of the heart, then that portion suffers an infarction—an attack—and dies. Sometimes the heart can survive such an attack and continue to perform its function, although the dead section turns a gray color and is called "ischemic."

For decades, surgeons have been inventing procedures to get at such occlusions, from reaming arteries out like a Roto-Rooter, to wrapping blood-starved portions of the heart with adhesive, hoping that the abrasion would force new vessels to spring up and serve the heart, to hooking up new sources of blood. None had proved satisfactory, but the search continued. The rewards were obvious, both in lives saved, and—bluntly—in potential patients. Some researchers hold that atherosclerosis is the body's natural aging process, that the occlusive building begins in late adolescence and can climax fatally at any time thereafter, if not elbowed out by cancer or infection or violence. A now-famous study of a large group of American soldiers killed in the Korean War revealed that up to 65 percent of these strong young men had recognizable atherosclerosis in their coronary arteries. This study exploded the belief that it was a plague of the aged.

Bingham's Phoenix cardiologist had run tests that indicated serious coronary artery disease and had dispatched him to Houston to see if Diethrich thought surgery was possible. Although DeBakey has built his reputation on the scalpel, he has also brought together all the medical disciplines interested in heart disease—chemists, biologists, radiologists, neurologists (for strokes), and cardiologists, who play the detective role and report to the surgeon what mysteries they have unraveled or suspect. They also recommended for or against surgery, which the surgeon may or may not accept. But in Houston the surgeon is, quite frankly, the Supreme Court.

At mid-morning, Bingham, wearing bright red-and-white striped pajamas, was wheeled by his brunette wife to Diethrich's cubbyhole office. There he learned that his first appointment would be with a cardiologist who wanted him to ride a bicycle.

Bingham, gregarious, bluff, overweight, hale-fellow-well-met, was obviously frightened but attempted to mask it with the bravado men use while taking Army physicals. There was a crater from an old football injury on half of his face. The cardiologist, Dr. Gerald Glick, appeared and said the test would take less than fifteen minutes, which put Mrs. Bingham at ease. Quiet, scholarly, Glick seemed the textbook image of the internist. Had it been the Middle Ages, the surgeons would have been out charging about on snorting steeds; the internists would have stayed in a secluded part of the castle reading manuscripts.

Glick led Bingham through a casual, but revealing, question and answer:

Q. "Are you married?"

A. "Happily."

Q. "Children?"

A. "Two, a boy 19, daughter 21."

Q. "What kind of work do you do? Is it a sedentary job?"

A. "No. I move around about 150,000 miles a year. I hire and train sales personnel. I guess you'd call me a professor of salesmanship."

Q. "You were in good health, you were well, until when?"

A. "Until about 1964. I got sick one day and it turned into pneumonia and I got over it and I went back to work full time. One night about midnight I was working and I felt this bad pain. It was like, ummmm, kind of like an upset stomach. Then I got the dry heaves and I couldn't throw up anything and I couldn't get comfortable. I spent all night draped over the toilet or tossing around in bed. It never occurred to me that I had had a heart attack, but my wife was worried and she called the doctor and it *was* a heart attack and they put me in the hospital for six to eight weeks."

Q. "Did you return to work?"

A. "Yeah. And six months later, I had what they told me was a minor infarction. That was March, 1965. I was hospitalized for only three days. Then these chest pains started."

Q. "What kind of chest pains? Can you describe them?"

A. "Sometimes it feels like an elephant is standing on my chest, pressing down with his foot."

Q. "Normally, what would bring them on?"

A. "That's the weirdest thing, Doc. I could go out and stand in a cold stream all day fishing, or hunting, or car racing—I'm one of the organizers and sponsors of the Phoenix sports car races—and it wouldn't bother me. But I could walk across my living room and the elephant would step on me again."

Q. "Some people can work all day and go home and see their wives and have angina pain."

A. "I don't have that problem. I *like* to see my wife."

Q. "Angina is caused by a simple imbalance between oxygen need and oxygen supply. The heart is not getting enough oxygenated blood, so it is, in effect, crying out. . . . These chest pains in 1965, were they your last complaint?"

A. "Just getting started. In December, '68, I had this pain all day long. I was conducting an eight-hour sales class. People told me later I looked bad the whole time. I was taking nitroglycerine tablets but the pain wouldn't stop. Finally I went to the hospital again for some relief and they slapped me right in ICU and I had an attack there. In the last six months the pains started coming two or three times a week, whereas it used to be only twice a year. My doctor in Phoenix, he told me that the way I live, the speed I go, he said he wouldn't give me much more hope."

Q. "Do you smoke?"

A. "Three, four packs a day. But I'm quitting."

Q. "You're a little overweight?"

A. "About 30 pounds. This bar in Phoenix put out a card listing all the qualifications to join the coronary club, the things you needed to do to *have* a heart attack, and I think I met every one of them."

Q. "Have any other members of your family had heart disease?"

A. "My brother had an attack when he was 35, one month after his wife committed suicide. And I have a sister who's the family hypochondriac. She has everything wrong with her; she had a heart attack when she was 47."

Q. "Approximately how long would a normal work day be for you?"

A. "Twelve, fourteen hours minimum."

Q. "Why did you come to Houston?"

A. "I heard about this new heart attack operation Diethrich's doing and I checked it out, and it seemed like this was the best place."

Glick put down his notebook and instructed Bingham to remove his pajama top and climb onto the white, Dutch-made cycling contraption. EKG leads were attached to his arms, and they in turn led to a monitoring device.

"We're going to measure your stress level," said Glick, in response to Bingham's inquisitive look. "We want to see at what level you begin to tire. We'll want to test you again three months after the operation. . . ."

Bingham interrupted. "Then I'm *going* to have the operation?"

"*If* you have the operation, then again in six months, then in a year."

While Glick checked the leads, Bingham talked on. "I told my doc in Phoenix that I wanted to come down here and get it over with. If I waited six months, then I might be dead—or chicken out."

He tested the pedals of the bicycle. "I could have brought my Honda and saved you all this trouble."

"But a Honda does all the work for you," said Glick. "Now just pedal normally and keep it up as long as you can."

Bingham began enthusiastically, moving the indicator up to 40 revolutions per minute. But after two minutes and 38 seconds he began to tire visibly, panting for breath, perspiring heavily.

Q. "Why did you quit?"

A. "I ran out of gas."

When Bingham left the room to go to another part of the hospital for his coronary arteriogram, the catheterization procedure, which can determine with remarkable accuracy exactly where the occlusion is occurring in the arteries, Glick wrote down his data. "Patients like Mr. Bingham think surgery is a great cure-all," he said, "that everything is fixed and that they can go back to leading the same old lives again at the pace which brought them here for surgery in the first place. I personally feel it is far too early to pronounce this new operation as salvation."

I remarked that many cardiologists seemed to be skeptical of the surgeon's activities.

"Not skeptical," he replied, "merely watchful. There have been so many of these great operations touted by the surgeons. There was one called the *poudrage*, which consisted of opening up the patient's chest and sprinkling talcum powder around the heart. The idea was that the powder would agitate the heart and cause it to form new sources of blood supply. It did no good at all, but it was popular for a while. Then there was one which was nothing but a mock operation. The patient arrived sedated at the operating room and there was a sealed envelope on the stretcher. The surgeon opened it—may I have the envelope, please?—and there were instructions from the internist on whether to do anything or *not* do anything at all. The patient never knew. He only knew that he had undergone a major operation on his heart by a great and famous surgeon. Strangely enough, it sometimes worked. The patient would find himself walking up a hill, a climb that would have given him terrible angina previously, and he would tell himself, 'I've just had an operation by a celebrated surgeon, so I won't get nervous and I won't have any heart pain.' This mock surgery pointed up the supreme importance of the doctor-patient relationship. If a patient has total confidence in his doctor, then often he is going to feel better, even if the doctor doesn't do much of anything—or nothing at all."

The Gypsy prince was better and receiving his family. I was escorted in by his son, a cheerful, corpulent copy of the father. About ten, he seemed as normal as any child that age when he spoke in English, but when talking with his father he slipped easily into Gypsy *patois*, an ancient language composed largely of Romanian and other mid-European dialects. Only then did a somewhat haughty cloak envelope him, he being of royal birth within the clan and heir to the throne or family roofing business or trailer, or whatever.

"This is my father," he said.

The stricken prince wafted one heavy arm in the direction of a chair. He was sipping orange juice and occasionally turned his head to watch the softly clicking monitor behind him, measuring his heart rate, and moving in steady, reassuring peaks and valleys.

"Perhaps we can arrange something," he said, answering an unasked question. "I have an incredible story which you could use. But it must wait until tomorrow." He spoke rapidly and quietly to his son in the Gypsy *patois.* "My son will introduce you to members of my family who will talk with you."

Two days after the bicycle test, Bingham was scheduled for surgery. The arteriograms had shown a definite blockage in the upper right coronary artery and quite probably the left; the flow of blood was severely reduced and there was no flow at all into one portion of the heart, which revealed an ischemic part from one of the past heart attacks. Diethrich had cautioned Bingham that the operation carried a fairly high risk, but that results on other people like him had seemingly been good. Overall, the mortality rate was less than 10 percent, but Bingham's heart loomed dangerous. He did not hesitate. "Cut," he said. "That's what I came here for."

In the doctor's dressing room I changed into a scrub suit and slipped green paper booties over my street shoes to ground them from producing sparks in a room where volatile fluids and oxygen would be used. Dr. Arthur Beall was talking with Dr. Reed, the young resident on duty in the Intensive Care Unit, the latter complaining mildly that he was losing weight and strength from the 30 days and nights he was spending there. Beall, a tanned, slender Baylor surgery professor with a marvelous Georgia drawl, could muster scant sympathy.

"In the old days," he said, recalling fifteen years before when he had been a resident under DeBakey, "The Professor had only one resident per 90-day period; he only wanted one because he didn't want a lot of people passing the buck, and we did *everything.* You only have ICU to worry about. My intern would throw cold water on my face at 5 A.M. and drag me out of bed, and I'd see 120 patients by seven o'clock. Then I'd go into surgery and first assist the Professor on about ten cases, which lasted all day, and in between I'd be slipping out and running ICU, working up new patients, making afternoon rounds from five to six, making secondary rounds after that to answer all the questions they couldn't ask DeBakey, writing medication, writing discharge reports, and getting to bed at 3 A.M. Only to get hit with that ice water at five. The average resident in my day lost twenty pounds."

Reed was listening in the manner of a child hearing his father tell of walking to school ten miles in the snow.

"The only thing that saved us from going batty," said Beall, who was not nearly done, "was the hospital telephone operator. When the Professor would go out of town, we'd slip home and see our wives for a few minutes, and if DeBakey called in from out of town, the operator would recognize his voice and put the call through direct to our home. He wouldn't know where we were talking from. One night this kid was home visiting with his wife and he got a call from the hospital saying that there was an emergency and he took off fast, only lived a few blocks away. It was shortly before midnight when he left and at 12:01 A.M. exactly, just before he reached the hospital, he got broadsided by a drunk driver. The next thing he knew there was a photographer there and the next morning his picture was on the front page of the paper because it was the start of Safe Driving Day and his was the first accident that day in Houston. Readers probably thought the young doctor looked so pained because of the accident, but the truth was he was imagining what DeBakey was going to say to him."

"Is that right?" said Reed.

Arthur Bingham had been sedated in his room, his chest hair shaved down to his belly button and his toupee removed. One of the EEG technicians who would monitor his brain waves explained the reason for the latter: "The toupee might get bloody, and because I have to stick three or four electrodes on the side of his head and if the toupee fell off during surgery, so would they." The brain waves are watched anxiously during surgery because it is possible for the patient to survive the operation but become the living dead if the brain's appetite for oxygenated blood is interfered with. More than a dozen probes were being stuck into Bingham—one in his neck, another for intravenous fluids, one to measure arterial pressure, one for venous pressure, a Foley catheter in his penis to remove and measure urine, one for temperature. He was beginning to take on the familiar look of the mechanical man when Diethrich entered the suite at 10:20 A.M., about half an hour after the preliminaries had begun. Ted looked down at Bingham, lying nude on the table. "He's a big brute, isn't he," said the surgeon to no one in particular. "He's got very bad heart disease." Two visiting surgeons from Holland had come in with Diethrich and he went over to explain the patient's case history and what he was going to attempt to do.

The anesthesiologist had Bingham well under by now, with a respirator machine breathing for him. He had been given 10 cc's of Innovar, a "miracle" narcotic. "The beauty of this stuff," said the anesthesiologist, "is that it does not bother the integrity of the cardio-vascular system at all. Nor will it depress the heart muscle. The only danger is that too large a dose given to a college-age kid might make him think fuzzily for a couple of weeks."

"Do patients ever remember anything about their operations?" I asked.

"We had one woman who was a poet and who claimed later to have total recall of everything—of the adhesive tape we put over her eyes, or being able to see the lights, anyway, of hearing the music come over the Muzak, of what Dr. DeBakey had said. She even wrote a poem about it. But I never believed her, she just had a good imagina-tion. Besides, we also give patients a drug called Scopolamine, which produces retroactive amnesia. Bingham here won't remember a thing; the next few hours are wiped out of his memory."

"Okay, everybody?" Diethrich's boyish Michigan tenor broke through the murmurings and the canned music. "Let's go." He glanced at the wall clock. It was 10:27.

Diethrich first cut into the fleshy inside part of the upper thigh, probing around about an inch from the surface until he located a large, sturdy-looking vein. He pulled it out, stubbornly, like wrestling a fish worm from the earth, and handed it to Hans Paessler, a young German doctor spending a non-credit year watching and helping out in Houston. Paessler dropped the vein into a metal dish and began flushing saline solution through it, both cleaning it and at the same time searching for tiny holes to sew up and make sure it was a leak-proof vessel.

Now the surgeon took a scalpel and sliced into the chest, from the neck to the point just above the navel, about fourteen inches in all. For a few unpleasant moments there was the acrid odor of searing flesh in the operating room as he cauterized the tiny blood vessels that fed the skin. Smoke rose from the wound. Melody,

Diethrich's scrub nurse, had the electric saw ready without being asked. The day before, she had scrubbed for Diethrich and the entire two-hour procedure was a mute, exquisite suite for four hands. Not a word had passed between them. "After you've done enough of these," said Melody, "you learn to stay at least one jump, if not two, ahead of your surgeon."

As a medical student at the University of Michigan, Diethrich had formed a surgical instruments company and invented the electric saw that he was now preparing to use. Placing the cutting edge at the top of the long incision, he gave a firm nod to the circulating nurse, who switched on a power source. Some surgeons use the saw and shake not only the patient, but the table, vibrating like a riveter working forty stories up on a naked skyscraper. But today the saw chomped smoothly through the tough breast bone.

Retractors were put in place to push back and hold the rib cage open, Diethrich snipped the pericardial sac, and the stricken heart was bared for all to see. An awesome sight! Almost gold, with patches of mauve and plum, there were criss-crossings of blue and black—a canvas of such color and form that DeBakey has been known to pause at this point of the operation and cry, almost religiously, to students: "Isn't this beautiful! Come and see the human heart!" On this morning Diethrich stopped as well, peering intently at the fist-sized object, a heart contracting and expanding almost indolently, annoyed, perhaps, at its first public exposure, a heart that had begun to grow and beat when the now massive Arthur Bingham had been but three weeks formed in his mother's womb and not yet as large as a thimble.

"I don't know what we can do," said Diethrich, who was rarely pessimistic.

(*"Before I came down here," Bingham had told me, "I went through a two-week period of thinking that I was not going to make it. I set things right with my business. I signed 'pending' contracts, made 'pending' deals, the 'pending,' of course, meaning my upcoming death."*)

Suddenly the heart seemed gross, threatening. Surely the surgeon would not invade it. He would sew the chest closed and. . . . But the moment passed. Diethrich began again, inserting the transparent tubes that would hook up the patient to the heart-lung oxygenating machine four feet from the operating table. This is the machine that gave birth to open-heart surgery in 1955. For the first time it allowed the surgeon to travel into the unknown, to, in effect, stop the heart, cut into it, and repair its defects.

The average human contains almost five quarts of blood, which is drained out through the tubing, flowing into the bypass machine, where it is oxygenated (the work of the lungs), passing back through tubing into the body. The cycle takes 40 seconds and is repeated continuously until the surgeon is finished and removes the clamp from the aorta—the "big pipe," largest blood vessel in the body. This allows blood to flow once again into the coronary arteries and nourish the heart muscle, provided, that is, the surgeon has not made a fatal blunder while working in its depths.

"Look at that!" cried Diethrich in alarm. He had slipped his latex-gloved hands gently beneath the now arrested heart. He lifted it and showed the Dutch surgeons that portion of Bingham's heart that had suffered the infarction. "The whole apex is ischemic," he said. "I don't think we can do anything for this guy."

(*"I'd rather die than be an invalid," Bingham had said. "The only thing I want is a few years of peace. My heart has aged my wife at least a decade. She's gone through more worry, strain, and stress than I did. It's ruined us financially. I was eating about $70 worth of pills a month, 24 pills a day for the past three years. All in all, it has cost me $20,000."*)

Hans had finished cleaning and leak-proofing the leg vein and brought it to the table in its metal bowl. He stood beside the surgeon and watched. Suddenly Euford Johnson, the bearded, bookish technician operating the oxygenating pump, said sharply: "Dr. Hans, don't lean on that cable. It's the patient's lifeline."

Hans side-stepped slightly and mumbled something inaudible in German.

"I hope," said Euford sweepingly, "that you are not resorting to sarcasm." Majesty and tension are sometimes present in the surgical suites; more often there is the routineness and bickering of any business anywhere. How could it be otherwise? Of 25,000 open-heart operations done each year in America's 7,000 hospitals, almost 10 percent are done in the two Houston institutes.

The surgeon ignored the sniping behind him and asked for the metal bowl. He clipped off a section of the vein about five inches long and began the most tedious and nerve-clenching procedure known to surgery, surpassing even the almost microscopic work done on the cornea of the eye. The job here was to sew one end of a vein into the aorta, the other end into the coronary artery buried within the heart—bypassing the area of occlusion. The surgeon must put up to twenty stitches across the mouth of the borrowed vein, an area approximately 1/25th of an inch across. It would be easier to sew twenty stitches into the end of a piece of spaghetti and affix it to a ripe pulsating pear. Some surgeons use magnifying loops attached to their eyeglasses so they can better see the infinitesimal sewing field.

If the operation works, the heart has a new piece of plumbing; it is revascularized. Blood begins flowing immediately into the thirsty, threatened part of the heart. Angina pain has been known to disappear immediately. The catch—a considerable one, the object of debate between some cardiologists and surgeons—is just how long the new pipe will stay open and unclogged. Presumably the condition within the body that caused the natural artery to block up will sooner or later repeat inside the new one. But how long?

(*"A man can live with this for the rest of his life, they tell me. And hell, life goes on. My kid's still in college, he needs money, the mortgage payments on the house don't stop when I have a heart attack."*)

For three quarters of an hour Diethrich sewed. His original plan was to do two bypasses in both the right and left coronary arteries, but he decided after the first was implanted that one would do the job. His mood turned rapidly to elation. "I think it's going to work," he said, and moments later, "in fact, it's going to be fantastic!"

But the surgeon's pride in his work was academic until Bingham was taken off the bypass pump. Only then would it be known if the heart was going to tolerate the reconstruction. Melody had defibrillating paddles ready in case they were needed. These are two metal disks used to provide a mild jolt of electricity. Sometimes, when a heart has been stopped by the surgeon and then allowed to start, it leaps up and beats in an undulating, erratic, jellyfish-like rhythm called fibrillation. Usually electricity can stop this dangerous rhythm and send it back to normal pulsation.

Diethrich ordered the pump shut off. Bingham's heart did not hesitate. It began to beat normally. The surgeon smiled behind his mask.

"Incredible," said one of the Dutchmen. The other made a small bow of appreciation. Diethrich stood beside his patient for a few moments, admiring his creation, then he was off to another patient waiting on another table. Hans Paessler and a resident would sew up Bingham's chest and escort him to the Intensive Care Unit.

I was hurriedly changing out of the greens into street clothes because I was late to a luncheon appointment. Two surgeons were changing as well, talking as they dressed of the new operation that Diethrich had done. "In five years," one of them said, "we'll be doing more of these than hernias."

"We'll all be blind, too," said the other.

At 3 A.M. the next morning, while the Gypsy's family slept fitfully on the chairs and floor of the sixth-floor waiting room, Prince Thomas suddenly seized his chest, gasped, and collapsed into unconsciousness. The floor nurse had peeked in on him minutes before and he had been resting calmly. On her next check, she was shocked to see the EKG monitor leaping erratically. The peaks and valleys had turned into erupting rockets. She paged Santiago, the Argentine surgical fellow on night duty, who came running into the room within 30 seconds. Instantly, Santiago saw that the Gypsy's heart was fibrillating. He worked on the huge body for more than an hour, jolting it again and again with the paddles—350 milliamps of electricity. He slammed his palms into the clammy, cooling chest, he plunged adrenalin into the heart, he fought until his forehead was drenched with sweat.

"He's not coming back," Santiago said. "The heart is completely arrested."

"He was fine earlier," said the nurse. "He drank his juice and talked to his family." She gestured with her head to the waiting room.

With a towel, Santiago wiped off the Gypsy's chest and head, then walked quietly down the hall. The clan knew. During the failing hour, one of the brothers had heard the clatter of running feet and the emergency cart rolling toward the prince's room and had followed. He had peeked through the crack of the door and saw the drama. Santiago had whirled and asked him to go away. Now the clan was sobbing and moaning in exotic grief. One ancient woman sang a dirge.

The brother demanded that the lights in the dead prince's room be left on until dawn, until the sun itself could wash the Gypsy, until an absent member of the tribe could be found to perform the rite of pronouncing death and transferring responsibility of the tribe to the little boy. Santiago nodded in agreement. He also permitted two of the old women to enter the room with lighted tapers and sit beside the body.

Early the next morning, Jerry Johnson asked the Gypsy's brother for permission to do an autopsy.

"What happened to my brother?" was the answer.

"Well, he died during the classic danger period I warned you about —that week to ten days following a heart attack. A piece of his heart probably infarcted, or 'died.' It was almost a rupture of the heart."

"But what caused his death, *exactly?*"

"We won't know *exactly* until we do a post."

"No. No. It's against our custom."

"Then," said Johnson, not pressing the point as ordinarily he would have done, "we'll never know."

That afternoon Santiago was in the bullpen recalling the experience. "Frankly I was scared to death," he said. "In my country, had this happened in the middle of the night with only one small doctor and one little nurse, the whole family would have turned on us."

"The Gypsy shouldn't have died," said a doctor on DeBakey's staff, later. "He shouldn't have left Kansas or wherever it was in the first place. He should have been slapped in a coronary-care unit there where they could watch him 24 hours a day rather than on a post-operative floor, and he should have been admitted under the care of a cardiologist. Certainly not a surgeon."

CHAPTER

3

After a quarrel with her estranged husband, followed by a yelling argument with her mother for an entire afternoon, a 23-year-old pregnant Houston cocktail waitress named Elizabeth Dagley locked herself in the bathroom in mid-April, 1970, shook out 50 Valium tranquilizer tablets into her hand, took every one of them, swallowed something else from another bottle she found in the medicine cabinet, and lay down to die. Her mother discovered her and phoned for an ambulance, which rushed the girl to Ben Taub General, the charity hospital for Houston and Harris County, named after De-Bakey's friend and benefactor. Ben Taub is located in the Texas Medical Center, connected by tunnel with the Baylor College of Medicine, and but a few hundred yards away from Methodist and St. Luke's Episcopal hospitals.

At first glance, Taub's Emergency Room seems a carnival of suffering, violence, and delay. At the admitting desk, mothers stand with feverish children slung whimpering over their hips, alcoholics tremble with DTS, children who have fallen out of trees or stepped on nails or pulled pans of boiling grease onto their heads, wait to be

treated by an exhausted but usually efficient team of residents and
interns from adjoining Baylor. Some women have learned to wait
until after 10 P.M. to bring their sick children in, knowing that the
pediatric clinic closes at that hour and that in the turbulence of the
Emergency Room, they can often get by without paying, and can
almost always get faster service. One of the duties of the poor is to
wait.

Several times each night and double that on weekends, people
whose lives have been very nearly destroyed by bullet or knife or
cars or their own hand are brought dying to Taub's Emergency
Room and hurried into one of two Shock Rooms. A team of fifteen
doctors and nurses swarm over the victim and within seconds have
intravenous fluids started in both arms, an airway, if needed, jammed
down the throat, bleeding stopped, vital signs measured, and on the
most desperate occasion have cracked the chest for emergency surgery. Every city should have Shock Rooms like these, manned by
round-the-clock teams, but they are an enormous expense to equip
and operate; most hospitals settle for those Emergency Rooms that
are all too often staffed by a nurse who is somewhere else in the
building when a case comes in and who has to telephone the doctor
"on call." Translated, that often means he is at home. Sick people die
every day while the nice woman from Admitting is asking questions
about Blue Cross and putting a plastic identification bracelet on
their arms.

When Elizabeth Dagley was wheeled into the Taub Emergency
Room, no questions were asked. The ambulance driver shouted "OD"
as he pushed the stretcher through the doors and a resident directed
the stretcher to the room in Emergency where overdoses are treated.
Two or three suicide attempts come in each night, but unless there is
great loss of blood, they do not have to go to the Shock Room.
Elizabeth, woozy but still conscious, confessed that she had taken 50
Valiums. "Anything else?" asked the tired young doctor. Elizabeth
shook her head negatively. She was given a drug to make her vomit
and her stomach was washed out, a messy, smelly process. A tube
was rammed down her throat into her stomach and water was pumped
down, 50 cc's at a time, then drawn back up with a suction machine,
repeated over and over until the water came up clear. An intravenous

was put in her arm to flood the body with fluids and step up urination, to pass out tranquilizers that might have reached her kidney.

But within a few hours, Elizabeth fell into a coma and started turning blue—symptomatic of barbiturate poisoning. She had also taken, it turned out, a hefty dose of phenobarbital but had not told the doctor about this. It was attacking her liver and brain. "There are two kinds of suicides," observed one of the residents. "Those who mean it, and those who don't. This old gal obviously meant it, or else she would have told us about the phenobarb." Elizabeth stayed in a coma for four days and on the afternoon of the fifth, her brain waves went flat. After a few hours, she was pronounced "brain dead" by a staff neurologist.

When a young, previously healthy, and—that curious medical term —"well-nourished" person dies, the nearest relative is routinely asked to consider donating organs to potential recipients who might be waiting. Elizabeth's distraught mother agreed and telephone calls quickly poured out to hospitals and medical centers in the area.

Did Galveston need an eye? A cornea? No.

Did Dallas have anybody worked up and waiting? Parkland Hospital there could use a kidney. Could Houston do tissue typing and fly it up?

Someone remembered that Howard Stapler was across the street at Methodist waiting for a heart; Ted Diethrich was notified. He felt Elizabeth's heart was worth studying for a possible match. He hung up the phone and hurriedly instructed his research nurse, Kem, to prepare the cardiac preservation chamber.

In 1967, when transplantation of hearts was still confined to dogs, Diethrich had found some research money and persuaded the Grumman Aerospace Corporation to put engineers to work constructing a machine about the size of a kitchen dishwasher. The idea was to remove both heart and lungs from a donor, put them into the chamber, bathe them with a cooling mist, keep them under constant monitoring, and preserve them alive and healthy until they could be transplanted into a recipient. The chamber had to be small and portable so it could be flown anywhere in the world. Several dog hearts had been kept alive for more than 30 hours, and on one occasion, in late 1969, a human heart had lived within the chamber for almost two days.

As a test, Diethrich even chartered a Lear jet and flew the chamber successfully to a hospital in San Antonio. To see the suspended organs pulsating within the chamber—the heart beating from its natural pace-maker—seemingly floating in the mist, was to think of the lab in a horror film. Diethrich took a lot of kidding as Dr. Frankenstein. He saw his project in a different light. "This is outer-space medicine," he said.

Stapler was not notified this stormy April late afternoon that the heart of a "technically dead" cocktail waitress was being considered for him. Twice before his hopes had been aroused, twice before the match had been deemed too poor to attempt. The results of heart transplantation during the years 1968 to 1969 had been so disappointing that only the best matches of donor and recipient were even being considered now. One of the other facts that nagged at Stapler's doctors was his morale: his decade of pain and sickness had left him addicted to morphine, had made him listless, had gravely depressed him.

The room was almost dark, and outside, rain swept against the windows in sheets. Stapler was dozing in his chair, a Western paperback open in his lap. When the door opened and the crack of light fell across his face, he opened his eyes. I started to leave, apologizing, but he called out. "No, no, come in. I'm not asleep. I was just reading. . . ." He held up the book. "I like the kind of stuff Ike used to read," he said. "And he fooled a few heart doctors in his time, too."

He got up slowly and eased his thin, unused body into the bed, gesturing for me to take his chair. He found a cigarette and lit it with a I-know-I'm-not-supposed-to shrug. "I was thinking of my home," he said. He did not turn on the light for a while and there were only the voices of two strangers and the glow of his cigarette in the room.

"It's a small town in Indiana, sort of an artists' colony, real rustic, the new buildings aren't very popular there. Even the new bank looks a hundred years old. We're old fashioned there. My kids read about juvenile delinquency and student protest and they say, 'Daddy, what's that?' "

There was an accordion-file folder of family pictures beside his bed and next to it, a stack of Polaroid color photographs. He dealt them out on the bed in front of him, a man playing solitaire with the images of his children. I wanted to tell him that two floors below men and women were preparing to study a dead woman's heart to see if it could fit into this ghostly white body. Instead I asked if he would tell me the history of his illness. His eyes almost brightened; for a few moments, as he spun his tale, they lost the film that had grayed them. He knew his story well, he had exact dates, hours, minutes of his multiplying catastrophes. It became apparent that his heart was the dominant factor of his life. It was his occupation. It was his obsession.

"On January 16, 1961," he began, "I was driving down the highway. I was in sales and promotion for heavy industrial equipment. Nice day. No ice on the road. I had both hands on the wheel and suddenly pain shot down both of them. I stopped the car and got nauseated and opened the door and vomited. I drove on after a while and I must have stopped a dozen more times. I finally got to a hospital in Franklin, Indiana, and four days later—a Sunday morning—I had a second heart attack. I spent four months there. They let me go back to work on July 1, and exactly thirteen days later I had a third heart attack in an Indianapolis hotel. This time I knew what was happening, so I drove myself to the Methodist Hospital. By April, 1965, I had had seven heart attacks.

"I went to one of the specialists in Cleveland and he examined me and condemned me to die. He gave me six months, a year at best. He said if I ever ran a dozen steps, I would meet my Maker. Well, you can imagine how many different doctors I must have talked to from 1961 to 1965, and I kept noticing that all of them would tell me different things. I started reading the medical journals and asked pretty good questions, and some of the damn doctors—pardon my French —didn't even know what I was talking about, much less know how to answer my questions.

"One afternoon in November, '65, I'd been to a cardiologist in Indianapolis and I'd picked up my heart catheterization report and I was driving down the I-65 and got a little tired so I stopped off at a roadside park. I was reading the cath, trying to figure out what it meant, and somehow—I'll never know the reason—the name De-Bakey flashed into my head. I had a $10 roll of quarters in my pocket. I decided to go for broke and call him. I found a pay phone and dialed Houston. He answered the phone himself. I gave him my case history while all the while dropping quarters in the phone. When I was down to fifty cents, he told me to come right on down to Houston.

"DeBakey operated on December 27, 1965, he went in and scraped the heart raw and implanted an artery. The next day my house burned to the ground in Indiana! My family didn't tell me about it for six weeks. They didn't want to excite me any more than I was. DeBakey's operation did some good, but by late 1966 the pain was back and so bad that DeBakey did another artery implant. I went home to Indiana and sat around and made a big mistake by reading about a new gas-jet operation they were doing in New York City. I asked around about it, and a doctor friend said if I went there and had it, I'd come home in a pine box.

"I had learned you shouldn't always believe doctors, so I went to New York City. And that was the biggest mistake I ever made. It was June, '68, and they did this new operation on me—they shoot little jets of carbon dioxide gas into the blocked-up heart arteries and pull out cores of blockage—and while I was still in Intensive Care, I got up goofy and walked out of the hospital and actually made it several blocks before somebody missed me and went out to look for me. When they found me, I was dragging bottles, IV tubes and squirting blood out of my femoral artery every time my heart beat. To top that, the new operation worked for about two weeks before the arteries clotted up again, and when I got home I was bedridden two months with infection."

Stapler took a long sip of ice water, but ignored the food tray that a dietician had brought in during his monologue. Could he eat the night of his transplant?

"From 1968 on," he continued, "I've had almost constant pain from angina; if you took a hammer and hit each one of my fingers, it wouldn't hurt more than it does now. DeBakey tried two months ago to do something else, but my heart stopped cold during the operation. Dr. Dennis, he's my cardiologist, he came out and told my wife he was extremely sorry but this time I was definitely dead. About 30 minutes later out comes DeBakey grinning and shouting, 'We did it! We did it!' But what he meant was that he had started up the heart."

But what were his thoughts about borrowing someone else's heart? The dice seemed to have only twos and twelves in them.

"I've already died four times," he said softly. "Once in an ambulance on the way to some hospital, somewhere, my heart stopped and the attendant beat on me with his fist so hard and so long that my chest was black and blue for months. I've got 75 inches of scars on my chest and there's nothing left but to try another heart. . . . I never thought I would die. I still have a little optimism left. My kids are too precious for me to leave. I've got a nice little wood-working shop to go home to and I'll make somebody some nice cabinets and tables."

He fell silent and I thanked him and started out. He stopped me. "Some day I'm going to be lying here in the middle of a Zane Grey and the nurse is going to come in and say, 'Okay, Howard, up and at 'em. There's a heart downstairs with your name on it.'"

As Stapler talked, Diethrich was at that very moment learning that Elizabeth Dagley had suffered severe pneumonia during the five days she lay comatose. Her heart was too contaminated by pneumonia to consider using it for transplantation. All Howard Stapler would receive this night would be a shot to kill his pain and a shot to put him to sleep. No sooner had the surgeon called off the cardiac preservation chamber than did the telephone ring again. This time it was Dr. Suki, a renal specialist at Baylor, asking if Diethrich could do a kidney transplant later that night. Diethrich agreed. He did not ask who the donor was, nor who the recipient would be. Not until a few moments before the operation began would he learn that the kidney had come from Elizabeth Dagley. Her heart was not suitable for a transplant, but neither of her kidneys had been affected by the pneumonia.

Two months before this, an eleven-year-old boy named Wesley Connor from Fort Polk, Louisiana, had been worked up by Dr. Suki, found to be a suitable candidate for a kidney transplant, and was told to stand by at his home. Wesley had been born with a chronic bladder condition, which had destroyed his kidneys; he had been urinating through two holes created near his navel, the urine flowing into pouches strapped around his waist. His mother and stepfather had bought a new car in anticipation of a sudden emergency summons. On the afternoon it arrived, they scooped up Wesley from a playground and were racing toward Houston.

The body of Elizabeth Dagley was transferred by ambulance the 1,500 yards across the Medical Center and she was wheeled into Room 3. The respirator was forcing her lungs to inhale and exhale; the illusion of life still clung to her. But her face was shut by death.

At 10:35 P.M. Diethrich scrubbed to go into surgery. Jerry Naifeh, the medical student, asked him what the case was going to be. "Kidney transplant."

"Who's the recipient?" asked Jerry.

"Some kid. I don't know him," said Diethrich.

"Who's the donor?"

"Cadaver. I'm just going to sew it in. This is the odd thing about transplant surgery; you don't meet the patients sometimes until you see them on the table."

Wesley was being prepared for surgery. A round-faced blond youngster with freckles, he had wide blue eyes stretched with apprehension over what was going to happen. Patients normally are sedated in their rooms before surgery so that they enter the operating room tranquil and sleepy. But Wesley had gone directly from his stepfather's new car into the operating room. A nurse was bent over him, gently talking nonstop, diverting his attention from the hot lights and the dozen people busied about him with needles, bottles, and tubes.

"Do you have a dog? Do you help your mama? Do you like to cook? Hamburgers? You seem like a 100 percent boy to me. . . ."

Wesley looked up and saw the off-duty nurses and students watching from the glass dome. A transplant always draws an audience. The nurse threw her hand over his eyes to block the sight but it was not necessary; the anesthesiologist had gone to work and the child's eyes closed quickly on their own.

It was almost midnight when Diethrich opened Wesley's abdomen and removed his kidney, a shriveled, useless organ. It was sent to pathology for examination and study. In the adjoining operating room, a resident had sliced open Elizabeth's stomach not quite so carefully and removed both of the kidneys. Mrs. Dietrich (no relation to Ted Diethrich) the head operating room nurse, put one kidney into a steel mixing bowl filled with saline solution and bore it cautiously to

Wesley's room. It had been carefully flushed with a solution to remove any blood clots and the tranquilizers and barbiturates that
Elizabeth had used to destroy herself.

Several doctors were around the table watching the transplant. "I
don't know how in hell Ted's going to fit that big kidney in that little
boy's pelvis," one of them said. The girl's kidney was approximately
twice the size of the one from the child that had been removed. The
doctor beside him drawled loudly, "I hope y'all washed the barbiturates out of that gal's kidney; you don't wanna put this little boy
to sleep forever."

Mrs. Dietrich bustled next door again to supervise the packing of
Elizabeth's other kidney for shipment to Dallas. The respirator had
been turned off and Elizabeth Dagley was forever dead. A resident
was stitching up her incision; someone had tied a tag with her name
on it around her toe. The color of death is blue if the breathing stops
first; if the heart stops first, it is gray.

Though she had been technically dead for nine hours now, Elizabeth was still building up a sizable hospital bill: the ambulance ride
across the Medical Center, the operating room fees, the surgeon's
charges. But Wesley's mother had agreed to pay for all of the donor's
expenses; it has become established hospital policy for the recipient to
bear the donor's charges.

Mrs. Dietrich had found a white styrofoam case about a foot high.
The kidney was put into a steel canister, floating in a solution of cold
saline and then into the styrofoam case. There was a slight argument
between the efficient, veteran nurse and one of the young doctors
about whether to use dry ice or real ice packed around the canister.
Mrs. Dietrich, who wanted a small amount of dry ice, pointed out
that it would not be proper to send Dallas a frozen-solid kidney.
"Hmmm. I guess you're right," said the young doctor.

"Who's going to take it up?" someone asked.

"Probably some Braniff stewardess in her flight bag," said someone
else.

Somebody stuck their head in the operating room door and said,
"No hurry. Dallas found a pilot who's coming down to get it."

Mrs. Dietrich dropped dry ice into the box, sealed it up, wrapped
it well with tape, and slapped a FRAGILE, HANDLE WITH CARE sticker
on top. Dr. Suki had prepared a letter with the tissue typing results,

which was Scotch-taped on the side. The box was carefully carried out to the operating room administration desk, where an assistant hospital administrator would watch it until the messenger came to take it to the airport.

Wesley's right colon had to be moved up a bit to accommodate the new kidney: the child gained exactly one pound during surgery. Seven hours later, a transplant team in Dallas sewed Elizabeth's other kidney into a young man.

The next afternoon in DeBakey's bullpen, Hans, the German doctor, was talking with some of the students and residents about transplants. In his country, Hans said, a flat brain wave is required for 24 hours before the patient is legally dead. "Here," said Hans, "as soon as the wave goes flat, they start transplanting."

DeBakey was back. He returned to a house full of patients. Polly Tovar, his admissions secretary, does not need his authorization to tell patients to come to Houston. She takes most of his long-distance telephone calls, notes the particulars of the case and the referring doctor's opinion, and makes a generally immediate appointment for the patient to enter Methodist on a given date. Surprisingly, it is not difficult to gain admission to DeBakey's service, nor is there a waiting period of seldom more than a few days.

On afternoon rounds DeBakey was in a good mood; most everyone he had operated on before his European trip was now ready to go home, stitches out, bags packed, hopes up. "I'm sorry to ask this, Dr. DeBakey," said one elderly woman, almost timidly, "but I sure would like to get out of here."

"Don't be sorry about that," answered DeBakey, beaming. "That's what we doctors like to hear."

He dismissed Stapler, telling him he could just as easily wait for a heart at home in Indiana. "It doesn't take long to fly here, does it?"

"Couple of hours," said Stapler.

"You go on home then, and we'll let you know just as soon as we might be able to do something for you."

Stapler nodded glumly. His disappointment was clear. A year earlier there would have been more enthusiasm to transplant him.

Diane Perlman was not tolerating the pain from her amputation.
Jerry Johnson had become concerned over pus at the site of her
wound and had mentioned casually that DeBakey would take a look
at it upon his return from Europe. Mrs. Perlman referred to this
while DeBakey was examining her. His face visibly tensed. Outside, he stood Johnson against the wall. "You don't know anything,"
he said. "You don't know enough yet to tell anybody when I should
see them."

Johnson had unknowingly committed a blunder that others had
learned in similar hard ways: be extremely cautious in communicat-
ing postoperative complications. Years ago, one resident even wrote
down three rules and passed them on to his successor. They were:

"1. If the complication is minor, treat it yourself, keep it to yourself, and pray that it works.

"2. If it is major, wait for the best opportune moment—it may
never come—to tell the Professor that the patient is infected or that
the graft is bleeding.

"3. If the patient dies, pray that the Professor is out of town."

DeBakey's attitude toward death was puzzling; no physician likes
to lose patients. DeBakey, however, took death as an intolerable almost personal affront to his skill, to his very being. On the rare occasion that patients died on his table, he would cancel the rest of the
day's schedule, stalk to his office, shut the door, lock it, and stay inside
for hours.

One prominent Houston surgeon remembers an incident that occurred a few years ago. The story sounds suspiciously apocryphal,
but the surgeon swears he witnessed it. "The quickest way to get
fired off the Professor's service was to have someone die on you in
ICU. He'd come in with storm clouds over his head and look at the
patient and after a long while he'd look at you and he'd say, 'I don't
understand this, Doctor. I gave this patient a perfect operation and
now he's dead. How could this happen?' Well, sometimes he was
right. Often complications were the fault of the younger guys,
but when a surgeon does as many operations as DeBakey does, you
cannot expect 100 percent recovery. One afternoon a resident was

on duty in ICU and it was a day when DeBakey was leaving on a long trip. Suddenly one of the patients upped and died. The resident was petrified. He had already done a few wrong things; this was a major crime. He knew DeBakey would be coming through on rounds just before he left for the airport. So he took the monitoring wires off the dead man and transferred them to the patient in the next bed. He dumped a lot of medication down the dead man's IV tube, made sure the respirator was working, and swore the nurse to secrecy. DeBakey came through on rounds, stopped at the dead man's bed, looked at the monitor. The resident murmured, 'He's doing about the same, Dr. DeBakey,' and DeBakey flew off. The moment he left the hospital, the kid disconnected everything and pronounced the guy."

DeBakey's transplant team did four more kidney transplants the same week Wesley received his. Baylor hurried out a press release claiming a world's record, five kidneys in five days. All were "doing satisfactorily."

Seven days after his bypass operation, Arthur Bingham was preparing to go home to Phoenix. His color was good, his eyes were clear, he yearned for a cigarette, but he had not smoked one even though his fist clenched when others did around him. Diethrich had pronounced the new artery within his heart to be working beautifully, maintaining a good flow of blood. Bingham could have posed as a testimonial to the new procedure. "The only thing bothering me is The Roadrunner in the next bed," he said, pointing to a middle-aged man asleep. "Last night he stood up in bed and started taking his clothes off and thrashing around and yelling, 'Let's get outta this cheap hotel.' Then he urinated in the wastebasket. He's an old bachelor, he told me, and he's scared and lonely."

The Roadrunner was Miles Vogler, a merchant from Denver, who had come to Houston complaining of severe pains in his legs. He could not walk very far without having to stop and rest. An arteriogram revealed occlusion in his lower abdominal aorta, and Diethrich recommended a Leriche operation—a bypass around the obstruction using a Y-shaped Dacron graft, where the aorta branched off to supply the legs with blood. Vogler listened attentively as it was explained where the graft would be implanted in the area above the groin, then beckoned for Diethrich to come close so they could talk confidentially.

"I've been a bachelor all my life," he said in a gravelly voice. "I'm 55, and I never really fell in love. My doctor back home told me my sex life was about over, but Doc, I can tell you it isn't. I went to St. Paul a while back and met this lady and we made love twice a day for five days. Now I ask you, does that sound like my sex life is over? What I'm getting at, Doc, I just don't want you to cut anything you don't have to."

Diethrich nodded seriously. "This procedure will help the circulation in your legs only," said Ted. "As to your sex life, I congratulate you. I promise not to hurt it, but on the other hand, I can't guarantee it will be any better."

Vogler bit his lower lip. A few moments passed. He began hesitantly. "Well . . . okay. . . . When do you wanna do it?"

"Tomorrow."

"That soon?"

"Why not?"

"I guess so."

Vogler was scheduled, but that very night he packed up his things, ran frightened out of the hospital and flew back to Denver. A nurse witnessed the flight and reported, "He looked just like The Roadrunner."

About a fortnight later, the Roadrunner came *beep-beeping* back into the hospital, almost knocked down the same nurse, scurried up to Diethrich and once more agreed to surgery. The surgeon scheduled him the first thing the next morning, "before he gets scared and runs out again." The operation was entirely successful, but Vogler was still mentally fuzzy from the anesthesia and his stay in Intensive Care Unit. "Sometimes it takes a few days for the older patients to get their marbles lined up again," explained an anesthesiologist.

Later that week, DeBakey did six beautiful operations, including an aortic arch aneurysm, impeccably excised and replaced with a

Dacron graft. This is DeBakey's specialty; had he never touched a human heart, his place in the history books would have been secure from this work alone. Before 1952, these insidious weaknesses any- where along the aorta would swell and eventually rupture—the classic lay description is that of a bubble in an inner tube—and, as one surgeon recalls, "There was nothing for us to do but sit around in the coffee room and make bets as to when the aneurysm in Room 306 would burst and die." There is confusion as to who actually did the first excision and repair of aneurysms—some claim DeBakey in the 1951–52 period, others claim Dr. DuBost of France slightly earlier, but there is no doubt that DeBakey became the foremost practitioner and preacher of the gospel. In the mid-1950s at national medical meetings, some surgeons would get up and say it was dan- gerous, reckless, and foolish to even attempt such surgery; others would stand and report a series of six or ten. DeBakey would rise and report a series of two hundred and fifty, with such spectacularly low mortality rates that those present would either draw in their breaths in surprise or express disbelief.

One Houston physician who has worked with both DeBakey and Cooley recalled those early years:

"Both men always reported such excellent results that their peers thought they were liars. They weren't out-and-out liars, but what you call an improved patient is a value judgment. You may cure a patient's headache but have to cut his leg off.

"Mike and Denton accepted every speaking invitation from every county medical society. Mike became known as fearless for tackling desperate situations, ruptured abdominal aneurysms. They rapidly had their referrals and they rapidly had the largest series of operations ever reported. Pretty soon the guy with the aneurysm in New York would ask his doctor, 'Who's the best surgeon in this field?' and the doctor would answer, 'I don't know who's the best but the guy who's done the most is Mike DeBakey.' And the parent with a child with a hole in his heart would ask his doctor in Seattle, 'Who's the best for this?' and his doctor would say, 'I don't know who's the best but the guy who's done the most is Cooley in Houston.' And they very rapidly outstripped the more experienced and better known. Neither man oddly has ever relied on local referrals. Cooley gets a few; DeBakey gets hardly any at all." Neither world-famous surgeon is greatly popular in Houston's medical community.

When Albert Einstein suffered a ruptured aneurysm in 1955, his doctor telephoned DeBakey, described the case, and asked if surgery was possible. "By all means," said DeBakey over long distance. "In fact, I will dictate what needs to be done." But Einstein, perhaps feeling his work was done, refused surgery and died.

A young surgeon named Don Bricker came to Houston in 1961 from Cornell and was astonished to discover how rapidly and efficiently aneurysms were done, and the scope of the cases. "I had been in New York City and there was only one surgeon there even attempting them, and he took five or six hours on a case, and the patient often died. I walked into DeBakey's OR and he's doing five or six cases a day, and he took an hour on each one at best, and most of them lived!"

As he neared 62, everyone said DeBakey was making a few concessions to age. Rarely did he operate alone, calling upon Ted Diethrich or George Noon more and more to first-assist, and because they were full-fledged surgeons, often they did more. He no longer scheduled surgery on Christmas Day. (On a Christmas not too many years back, DeBakey was making rounds when he suddenly stopped to complain, "Where are all the residents? Where are all the interns and students? Nobody wants to help me; nobody cares anything about medicine any more." The resident accompanying him said, "Sir, they're all at home celebrating the birth of another great man." And DeBakey laughed.) Sundays were usually free now, but not always. Last year a DeBakey patient had been scheduled for an aneurysm operation on a Tuesday when suddenly one Sunday morning while sitting up in his bed he ruptured. DeBakey rushed him to the operating room, lost him, and then told his resident John Russell that he was going to operate on every aneurysm in the house. By late Sunday night he had done three or four, and none was in further danger of rupturing.

There was open gossip that the eyes looming so large behind the trifocals were not as strong as once they were; for that reason, people said, he did not attempt the spectacular but optically grueling coronary artery bypass. But on this April day, as he sliced and sewed in an aortic valve into the heart, as he beckoned for a visiting surgeon to come closer and look, it would have been difficult to fault any part of the man or his work. He operated as surely as any master craftsman. He grumped twice about his assistants, saying "Can't we do this right? For God's sake, haven't we done it enough?" And later, "If I only had a third sterile hand. . . . With a third hand I could do it all myself!" But these were outbursts, only minor rumblings, and they had been heard a thousand times before.

DeBakey had come to lean heavily on those who had been with him for many years, in particular two women. One was Mary Martin, the chief pump technician who had turned down an offer to go across the way and work with Cooley. In the beginning Mary had been the only pump technician; there were several now, but DeBakey called them all "Mary." During the operation he said, without looking behind him, "How are we doing, Mary?" and Euford, bearded, replied, "Just fine, Dr. DeBakey." The other woman was Ellen Morris, his personal scrub technician, the only one who ever scrubs for DeBakey. Each morning she rose early to pile her dyed blond hair up into an elaborate, towering coiffure, which she displayed beneath a see-through surgical turban of her own design. Other nurses had followed suit, and while most operating room women in hospitals elsewhere squashed their hair under flat, floppy caps, the women who worked on DeBakey's service looked as if they had just left the beauty parlor as they passed the needle holders and sutures.

Both Mary and Ellen were not only capable and dependable, but intensely loyal—defensive of DeBakey against a hint of criticism. When a reporter asked Ellen if it were true that he sometimes yelled at inefficient nurses, she replied: "Dr. DeBakey would never do that. He is, after all, a Southern gentleman."

On rounds that afternoon, Diethrich saw Mrs. Matthews, a tiny, wispy Florida woman on whom he had done two bypass arterial grafts, stretching practically from her armpits to her knees. She was a nice, uncomplaining lady, but one of those patients to whom complications swarm; every doctor has one disaster area like her on his service. She was in a special isolation room in the Intensive Care Unit for patients with infections. She reached up and took the surgeon's arm and pulled him down and whispered, crying, into his ear. He put on a false bright face and whispered back, patting her gently.

He went out and motioned for Dr. Reed, the resident in charge of Intensive Care, to follow him down the hall out of earshot. At about fifteen feet Diethrich whirled and anger erupted. "Have you ever been sick, Doctor?" he almost shouted, and, not waiting for an answer, "Would you like to be told you're bleeding internally?"

"But she was, she is," said Reed quietly, not used to seeing Diethrich this way.

"Good God, Doctor, you've got to reassure the patient. This is a nut house anyway! Don't make things worse. All you have to tell the patient is that she's getting the best care she can get. That's *all!* Understand? You're playing God! You can scare a patient to death, because they *will* die of fright. It can happen, I assure you, it can happen."

Bingham and The Roadrunner were both well enough to leave the hospital; Diethrich gave them a pass to spend a night on the town. They dined together at a seafood restaurant near the Medical Center and vowed—as people do on long ship crossings—to stay in touch.

Howard Stapler flew back alone to Indiana. But he had been there only a few days when a call came from Diethrich to prepare for a quick return to Houston. A hospital in Detroit had telephoned with a promising donor heart. A Lear jet was to fly there with the preservation chamber and pick it up. But within a few minutes, Detroit called back and the plan collapsed. The heart was a homicide case, and the legal complications were too tangled to unravel in the required speed.

Diethrich called the elated Stapler and told him to forget it for the time being. There was silence for a moment, and then both men hung up the phone.

CHAPTER

4

In the history of medicine, the surgeon waited a long time for
celebrity and the time when hospitals would be built around him.
The surgeon was considered an eccentric and second-class member
of the profession well into the twentieth century. He was put in
a special category and not permitted to associate with accepted
members of the profession. The surgeon's trade historically consisted of those patients who had been victims of violence; cutting,
probing, and sewing them up was hardly as sophisticated as the mysterious work done by physicians who diagnosed ailments and whose
shelves were crowded with pills and potions.

The art began in Egypt, as did most things, with certain people
whom the royal physician permitted to sew up stab wounds and
bind them with strips of cloth. A few centuries later in India, surgeons ventured upon the idea of taking a person whose stomach had
been gutted with a knife or a sharp pole and washing out the wound
with milk and rubbing it with butter. The real novelty of their treatment, however, was then letting black ants walk around for a few
days within the wound before closing it.

Pope Calistas, whose twelfth-century spiritual stewardship was not theologically noteworthy, nonetheless earned his place in medical textbooks by forbidding priests to attend the sick, a task they had previously monopolized. Who should take their place as bleeders and stitchers of minor wounds but, of all people, the barbers! These fellows not only had sharp blades to begin with, they also found biblical justification for their work in Ezekiel 5:1, "And thou, son of man, take thee a barber's razor. . . ."

The invention of gunpowder in the fourteenth century gave surgery its greatest impetus. As soon as men learned how to shoot holes into their fellow men, a whole new line of work sprang up for the barber-surgeons. They made sure that they would attract potential customers to their shops by rigging up poles outside splashed with blood and wrapped around with bandages (the ancestor of today's barber pole). Those legitimate surgeons who had been to medical school were so limited in their knowledge and skills that they offered little competition. A respected Italian surgeon, Giovanni da Vigo, for example, treated his gunshot victims by pouring boiling oil on the wound, followed by a plaster concocted from worms, minced-up toads, and snakes. A century later, a French surgeon, Dr. Paré was about to pour boiling oil on a wound—this being the accepted treatment of choice—when he discovered to his chagrin that his supply was depleted. He hurriedly brewed up a potion of oil of rose, turpentine, and egg yolk, and to his surprise, the patient healed faster than those who had received the burning oil.

For more than 700 years, barbers clung stubbornly to their knives, resisting the efforts of legitimate practitioners through the law and royal decree to wrest the privilege from them. Bloody battles were fought in the cobblestone streets of seventeenth-century Paris between barbers—who used the same *rasoir* for cutting off toes *and* trimming mustaches—and those doctors trying to establish a legitimate surgery within the Royal Medical Academy. But Louis XIV was so enthralled with his barber-surgeons that he ordered public demonstrations of surgery to be given on fair afternoons in the royal gardens. Fashionable citizens flocked to attend. Meanwhile, across the Channel, Henry VIII had granted a royal charter in 1540 to "The Masters, Guvernors of the Mystery and Commanlty of Barbours and Surgeons of London."

One of the few legitimate surgeons of Medieval times, a Frenchman named Henri de Mondeville who practiced at the beginning of the fourteenth century in Paris and traveled with the king and his armies, set forth four qualifications for a surgeon: he must not be afraid of evil smells; he must cut or destroy boldly—as an executioner; he must know how to lie in a courteous way; and he must know how to extract a gift or a fee from his patients.

Not unpredictably, other laymen tried to enter what had become a highly lucrative line of work. (One Paris barber-surgeon had an estate outside the city with 175 servants and stables for 300 horses.) In Copenhagen, the Danish king authorized the public executioner to do surgery when he was not otherwise engaged. Frederick I of Prussia in 1796 appointed his favorite hangman to be not only a public surgeon for the nobility, but his personal court physician. In Italy the steam-bath keepers so pestered the barbers for work that they finally were taken in as co-cutters. This news quickly reached Germany and Sweden, where the rich tradesman could, in one convenient visit, take steam and have a worrisome skin tumor sliced away. In nineteenth-century Austria, there still existed three classes of surgeons: doctors of surgery, medico-surgeons, and bath keepers. In Britain even today, the surgeon traditionally does not bear the title "Doctor." He is called "Mister," which must frustrate some parents who have paid for ten years of medical education.

What pulled the surgeon out of the barber shop and into the hospital were the advent of (1) anesthesia, in America, in the mid-nineteenth century, and (2) the use of sterile methods to fight infection, preached first by Lister in England, then by W. S. Halstead in America. Halstead, the great Harvard teacher and surgeon, introduced surgical gloves in 1890, *not* so much to protect the patient from possible infection, but to protect the hands of his scrub nurse, which had become chapped and rough. By 1911, masks were widely used, though some surgeons felt them unnecessary. Some general practitioners, however, agreed that the surgeon had at last chosen something that fitted his avocation, which bore a striking resemblance to the work of an executioner.

The conflict between physician and surgeon is as old as medicine and will endure as long as there are those who cut and those who diagnose. I once attended a patient conference at a medical school and the internist in charge, presenting the facts of a case, said matter-of-factly, "This patient was *subjected* to surgery." The phrase is heard in classes every day. One Houston heart surgeon, discouraged over a patient's death, remarked—not entirely facetiously—"The cardiologist kept this guy on the string for twenty years treating his angina; it was almost an annuity. When he finally went into massive heart failure, the cardiologist sent him to me at a minute to midnight." The internist would probably have snapped back, as I have heard other internists do, "It is my duty to protect my patient from the surgeon as long as possible." Eight hundred years ago, the French surgeon Mondeville wrote a treatise on his craft that drew the lines remarkably well:

"Surgery undoubtedly is superior to medicine for the following reasons:

"1. Surgery cures more complicated maladies, such as toward which medicine is helpless.

"2. Surgery cures diseases that cannot be cured by any other means, not by themselves, not by nature, not by medicine. Medicine indeed never cures a disease so evidently that one could say that the cure is due to medicine.

"3. The doings of surgery are visible and manifest, while those of medicine are hidden, which is very fortunate for many physicians. If they have made a mistake, it is not apparent, and if they kill the patient, it will not be done openly. But if the surgeon commits an error while performing an incision on the hand or arm, this is seen by everybody present and could not be attributed to nature nor to the constitution of the patient."

Mondeville then talked about the difficulty of getting work: "Even in the case of a strictly surgical disease, if a sly physician has been called first, never will a surgeon see the case. More than that, the physician will tell the patient, 'Sir, it is evident that the surgeons are vain and pompous people. They don't know anything about reasoning and are completely ignorant. If there is anything they know, they got it from us, the physicians. They are bad and cruel people, and ask for and receive huge fees. On the other side, you, sir, are feeble, inclined to be sick and delicate, and the expense involved in calling a surgeon could affect you too much. Therefore I advise you, in your interest, and out of sheer love, not to call for a surgeon, and although not a surgeon myself, I will endeavor to help you without them.' "

The Houston surgeon Don Bricker will have much to discuss with Mondeville if they ever meet sometime in a celestial medical society. "The surgeon," says Bricker, "is a therapist who wants to make the patient well. As contrasted with the internist, he wants to do it with his own hands. The surgeon doesn't seek the intellectual challenge which delights the internist. If a patient comes in with a hernia, he points to it, the surgeon recognizes it, the surgeon fixes it, the patient says, 'thank you.'

"The internist, conversely, gets his greatest satisfaction out of diagnosing some disease like Hodgkin's. The surgeon would be dismayed because he couldn't treat it. The surgeon is straightforward and lacks the deviousness of the internist. The internist is often bitter because the surgeon does not need him. The surgeon is the only member of medicine who is the complete doctor. There is no disease that isn't likely to develop someday into a surgical condition."

But there are two widely recited slogans in the medical schools of America. One, according to the internist, is the surgeon's motto: "When in doubt, cut it out." The other, which I saw on a Baylor students' bulletin board, is: "The surgeon's hands are lean and nimble; his head would fit inside a thimble."

A conversation with a Houston surgeon *not* affiliated with either Michael DeBakey or Denton Cooley:

Q. "Would you characterize the nature of the modern surgeon for me?"

A. "You can usually spot them in the first year of medical school. As a rule, the surgeon is the most well-coordinated individual. He's probably the best athlete, he is more gregarious, he's more affable, he's less introverted, he becomes more politically active, he is more ambitious. . . ."

Q. "You left out loyal, obedient, trustworthy, and brave."

A. "Those, too. As well as slightly egomaniac. But I would say to that, spare me the surgeon who doesn't have this ego. The man who cuts on you has to feel that he is the only man who can do the job. There is no room for weak sisters in the OR."

Q. "Would you say that DeBakey and Cooley are typical surgeons?

A. "Carried to the nth degree. Mike came to Houston in 1948
with a pretty fair country reputation as a cutter. He had been over
in New Orleans working for Dr. Alton Ochsner and he was very
much the junior man there. He was anxious to start running his own
show. What he found was medicine of an almost primitive sort being practiced here. He found none of the things they had promised
him in order to get him over as head of Baylor's surgery department. Baylor itself had only just been lured down a couple or three
years earlier from Dallas by a group of fat cats who coughed up
$10 million to get it here. Mike set things in motion from the first
week he arrived. For the past 25 years he has bludgeoned his way to
where he is, without doubt, the most powerful doctor in America.
When I talked to him in those days at first I thought he was a
megalomaniac—but now I realize he knew where he was going all
the time. He seemed to have a master plan even then. He let me
know in no uncertain terms that he—and what he was going to do in
medicine—was something special. He had a manifest destiny. But
then, in 1951, along came Denton Cooley, and so did he. Denton
had the same overview of history."

Q. "What was their relationship in the beginning?"

A. "Professional. No warmth. Mike, after all, had come from
a Lebanese immigrant family in Lake Charles, Louisiana, and his
mother taught him how to sew his own underwear and he worked
in his father's drugstore and when he finally got to Tulane, he was
not popular. In fact, he was very much an outsider, the owl, the for-
eigner, the guy who didn't get invited to join a top fraternity. It
wasn't that he was not well liked, I just don't think people paid much
attention to him at all. Cooley, on the other hand, was the son of a
rich society dentist in Houston and they owned a lot of the north side
of town. Denton was always the most popular kid in the crowd, the
leader, the one with charisma, the star athlete, the one all the fra-
ternities at the University of Texas fought to rush. And the hand-
somest son of a bitch to ever pick up a scalpel. How'd you like to
shave Mike DeBakey's face every morning and then have to look
across the table at Denton Cooley?"

Q. "Was there trouble between them from the beginning?"

A. "No. For a few years, Mike was the maestro, Denton played the protégé, although he was equally as skilled and knew far more about heart surgery—such as it was—than Mike. DeBakey, in fact, didn't start poking around hearts until about 1961. He had concentrated on his aneurysms and vessel work, Denton did the hearts, and the arrangement seemed ideal. I was around during the first big aneurysm DeBakey did, but not having the overview that he has, I didn't even know history was taking place. Judging from the coolness with which they went at it, you'd have thought it was a routine operation. Denton 'first-assisted,' but I heard, had you stood at the table, you might have wondered who was leading whom."

Q. "Why is there antagonism toward the two men within the Houston medical community?"

A. "Some are jealous. Hell, Mike and Denton shouldn't be doing hernias and gall bladders, but they do, and it is irritating to the rest of us. The patient is usually some prominent fellow who has asked for them and who might make a big donation to their causes. Others of us feel that medicine should be conducted quietly, privately, not in headlines or on the Johnny Carson Show. And with Mike, it's just because he is so impossible to deal with."

Q. "Meaning?"

A. "Meaning he is *consumed* with his work and himself. The human factor is missing. If you looked back over the careers of the great surgeons—and Mike is certainly in that category, it's tragic that his personality clouds his magnificent contributions to the art—you will find that all of them, Cushing, Halstead, whoever, had a peak period of perhaps ten productive years. These were years of impact. Of history. And then they de-accelerated, usually by more and more teaching, by developing rapport with their younger men, by helping them get good jobs and by taking pride in their achievements. There is none of this warmth, this fatherly feeling with Mike. Out of 25 years of heading Baylor's surgical department, Mike does not have one—not even *one*—chairman of a surgery department somewhere. Dr. Alfred Blalock, who was Denton's mentor at Johns Hopkins, has them scattered all over academic medicine. This is Mike's shortcoming—he becomes a rival to his own doctors. If he doesn't fire them or run them off, he becomes jealous and envious of them."

Q. "But what does the medical world as a whole think of De-Bakey and Cooley?"

A. "No matter what excesses they have committed, they have made Houston the finest cardiovascular institution in the world. We have doctors coming here from the seven continents to see in one week what they wouldn't see in years of observation somewhere else."

Q. "Is heart work done in Houston that is not done anywhere else?"

A. "No. Mike and Denton just do ten times more of it."

Q. "May I ask a rude question."

A. "Sure."

Q. "Are you ever jealous of those two across the street?"

A. "Truthfully? Of course. I sit here in a little office and Mike and Denton are over there in surgical palaces. But I content myself with knowing that I am a good surgeon, that I stay with my patient before, during, and after the operation, that I have a good relationship with my family, that I have a good relationship with my peers."

Q. "What is that peer relationship?"

A. "In Houston it is clean-cut. We are not a city brushed with sophistication. In New York, I know of internists who make sweetheart deals with surgeons. No one has ever spoken to me this way in Houston. If one did, the conversation wouldn't last fifteen seconds."

CHAPTER
5

Toward the end of April, 1970, a green, tropical month in Houston, Dr. Denton Cooley, then 49 years old, flew to a medical meeting in West Virginia where he concluded his speech by talking of his dormant transplant program. He defended his implanation of 21 human hearts and one artificial heart, illustrating his words with slides that showed groups of his transplanted patients, seemingly radiant with health, photographs taken before they began falling, one by one. The audience applauded not only the speech's content, but its delivery—low-keyed, boyish, earnest, Texan. It was a speech he would give several times in the months to come and invariably it would be successful. Cooley is not only a surgeon, not only a speaker, but a presence, frankly sexual. He accepts center stage as Olivier does, a possession earned. He rises slowly, unfolding the lanky, muscled body, walking with athletic grace to the lectern, pausing for a calculated second to meet the audience with his gray-blue eyes, and leads audiences into the awesome valley of open-heart surgery.

It may be facetious to talk of a surgeon by commencing with his looks but everyone does. One Houston matron, explaining her hypothetical choice of Cooley over DeBakey, said, "When I wake up from anesthesia, honey, I want Denton Cooley leaning over my bed." A Houston medical writer feels the physical characteristics are a major factor in aligning support within her city. "DeBakey, whom I feel is a deeper man, a more introspective man, nonetheless looks as if he could play Shylock," she says. "Cooley is the golden boy."

When Methodist Hospital and St. Luke's Episcopal Hospital were first planned in the early 1950s, the governing boards decided to specialize in different fields. After all, they were neighborly institutions only one hundred or so yards apart, and religiously endowed neighbors at that. In addition to general hospital services, Methodist would feature a psychiatric floor, orthopedics, a renal service, and neurological specialists. St. Luke's would handle urology and premature infants. Neither hospital made room for heart-surgery patients, because in the early 1950s there were none. Nor could the planners have foreseen the tidal waves of patients that would wash in from all over the world. Each hospital soon had to make urgent accommodations to stay up with the burgeoning heart business. Methodist, DeBakey's hospital, made four major additions, growing from an original size of 301 beds to its current 1,021, and added its spectacular Fondren-Brown wing. Cooley's St. Luke's moved more slowly but with a Texas-sized goal in sight. By mid-1970, a 27-story tower addition had been topped off, dominating the Texas Medical Center as the Colossus dominated Rhodes. There would be seven full floors for Cooley's Texas Heart Institute. Cooley had hoped to have the Institute in its new quarters by 1969, but labor strikes and a shortage of borrowable money had delayed it two years.

Houston is a rich city and its millionaires have become accustomed to answering the knock at their door and encountering DeBakey or Cooley or the head of another medical institution standing there with hat in hand. Dr. R. Lee Clark, who heads the massive M. D. Anderson cancer hospital across the street from Methodist and St. Luke's and who has plans to double its size, never loses his optimism. "I spent quite some time in Florence trying to see what brought about the Renaissance," he said one day as he showed me the table-top model of the additions. "I came to the conclusion that it was due to the people of the city and the scientists of the city working together. We're going through a Renaissance of Health in Houston. We've got people who aren't afraid of raising $100 million. Houston is a place where you can go and present an idea at dinner time and raise $3 million by 10 P.M."

Physically joined to St. Luke's Hospital with common corridors is the Texas Children's Hospital. When Cooley had grown disenchanted with DeBakey in the mid-1950s he had moved, without a formal break, to Texas Children's, where he began a series of heart operations on children. The hospital, one of the most remarkable in the world, had been funded in a manner unique, if not to Florence, then to Houston. Leopold Meyer, a wealthy Jewish merchant and developer, was enlisted to scout the city for money. He went to visit his Episcopalian friend, J. S. Abercrombie, who on the occasion of the visit was in a downtown Baptist hospital with a back problem.

"Say, Jim, you got any money?" asked Meyer after the social amenities.

"Little."

"Well, I want to spend some."

"What for?"

"We want to build a children's hospital." Meyer explained the idea and the potential.

"I'm not sure your idea is a practical one, but if you're that sold on it, how much money you talking about?"

"Couple of million dollars."

"Go ahead."

"I'm going to commit you, Jim."

"I know it. Now get out of my room. My back hurts."

Abercrombie later announced that he was tired of being solicited every year thereafter to make up the deficit of operating the hospital, so he pledged his dividends and stock holdings in the Cameron Iron Works for the next 40 years. "Our hospital," said Meyer, "will never be in want."

On the first Monday morning in May, 1970, Dr. Robert Leachman was holding forth in the Cardiology Section of St. Luke's, where he was the chief, trying with no success to get out and see the new batch of patients who had checked in the night before. In the two Houston hospitals, it is the problem of the cardiologist to dwell in the shadow of the surgeon—Leachman describes his role as that of "surgical pimp"—but he, in fact, seemed a good counterpart to the dash and élan down the hall. He had hair he had forgotten to cut, a suit he had forgotten to press, shoes he had forgotten to shine. A cigar seemed permanently growing on his hand or face, except on those reluctant occasions when he had to put it down on a window sill to enter a patient's room. His teeth were uneven, with a prominent gold one sparkling in front, but he was a man of gentle nature who, after being around for a while, became highly attractive. He was the country doctor in the city, but he was comfortable in the role. He spent as much time in the patient's room as the patient wanted; he never seemed in a hurry. He would lean against a staircase wall for half an hour to go over a puzzling EKG with a group of foreign cardiology fellows who trailed him. He was a philosophical, self-searching physician who fretted now and then that a surgeon got $1,500 for the operation that took only a half hour of his time, while a cardiologist billed a patient only $300 for managing him before, during, and the ten days to two weeks after the procedure.

Leachman spoke fluent if atrociously accented Spanish, which was valuable to Cooley because of the volume of patients streaming in from Mexico and South America. When the earthquake of 1970 devastated Peru, Leachman spent almost a week on the telephone trying to arrange to go there to care for the injured; the trip was never made because Peruvian authorities said they had enough doctors.

It took Leachman more than an hour to leave his office: three patients were waiting for catheterizations of their hearts, one woman from Long Island repeating over and over again, "I dread this more than I do surgery. For God's sake, knock me out." Leachman picked up her wrist and held it as if checking her pulse; doctors frequently do this and do not even bother to count. Pulse-taking can be a gesture of friendship and interest. "It isn't exactly painless dentistry," he told the woman, explaining that general anesthesia was not necessary, "but we try." A problem had arisen with a Spanish patient and three doctors—one from Venezuela, two from Mexico—were loudly debating it. Phones were ringing, the radio was turned up loudly to a rock and roll revival, the coffee pot was breaking down, a new secretary was breaking in, the air-conditioning system was out, a drug detail man was following the doctors about with a new pain-relief pill, and a two-year-old child, back for a postoperative checkup, was screaming, spitting out his pacifier, growing increasingly angry, finally throwing up on his mother, himself, a nurse, and the floor. Leachman looked slowly around and said quietly, "I think it's a good time to make rounds."

Cooley normally has from 80 to 100 patients in St. Luke's and Texas Children's, and he arbitrarily assigns each of them to a staff cardiologist. Leachman carries about 30 on his census. By the time a heart patient gets to Houston, he has been through the medical mill. If he is from a small town, he probably started with the local general practitioner, who, upon suspecting something wrong with his heart, referred him to the nearest big-city internist, who, if the diagnosis indicated surgery, dispatched him to Houston and Cooley.

"I've noticed there are two groups of patients," said Leachman as he ambled easily down a hallway. He had thrown his brown suit jacket over his hospital greens. I cannot recall ever seeing him with the crisp white glamorous coat that marks his profession. "There are the ones who identify instantly with the surgeon, and a second group which identifies with me. These are usually people who have been kicked around so long by their sickness that they know the surgeon is not the only answer."

Leachman was on the seventh floor of Texas Children's and he stopped at a nursing station to pick up a new patient's chart. Putting his smoldering cigar down on the edge of a new white formica-topped desk, he received a frown from the head nurse.

Leachman flipped through the chart. It told the medical history of a four-year-old child from Austin, Pamela Kroger, who had been born with the great vessels of her heart transposed. Until half a dozen years ago, such transposition meant early death, usually within a few weeks after birth. Now surgical correction is possible, done in two stages. In the first few weeks or months after birth, the infant receives a palliative operation to improve oxygenation. The surgeon, in effect, creates another defect to replace the primary one. When the child is four or five years old and better able to tolerate major surgery, total correction can be attempted. A Canadian surgeon, Dr. Mustard, was the first to carry out this procedure, but Cooley has since done more "Mustards" than all the other heart surgeons in the world put together. After a few months in Houston, the superlatives—the "more than's" and the "most of's" become familiar, even wearisome to the ear.

Leachman had said surgery was not the only answer to heart disease. How, then, had two surgeons built two heart centers in the same city, casting the cardiologist in a supporting role?

"Like it or not," Leachman said, "structural power, economic power, and political power rests in the surgeons' hands. They are not the intellectuals of medicine, but they have the clout."

He stopped and looked back at the nursing station. He was going to talk a while and he missed his cigar. "I'm not so sure I disagree with this, either. There needs to be a God-image. The patient has to have it all built up in his mind that this one guy and his two hands —that after all the other doctors who have pawed him and pulled him, after all the pills, all the pain, that this pair of hands is going to make him well. I would be uncomfortable thrust in the role of Super-Jesus, but somebody must play it. There is a well-known heart clinic in Mexico which decided to have a lot of important apostles and no Super-Jesus, and I believe it is about to collapse."

The transposition case, Pamela Kroger, began to shriek the moment Leachman entered her room. She was a thin, pale child with a bluish cast to her body. There was enormous pain and sadness in her presence, despite the dolls and laughing clowns scattered on her bed covers. The room itself was gaily decorated with one red wall and stylish lithographs of children and animals.

"Hello, Pammy," Leachman said, trying to take an unwilling pulse. He surrendered and pressed his stethoscope against her night-gown. Doctors who deal with children learn to listen patiently and catch the heart sounds in between sobs. Mrs. Kroger attempted to calm her child, but Leachman shook his head that it was not necessary. He motioned for her to follow him into the hallway.

"The catheterization tells us it's worth trying," he began. Mrs. Kroger nodded, biting her lip. "But there is, you should know, a definite risk involved." Mrs. Kroger nodded again; she was clutching her elbows tightly. "I suppose," Leachman said, "everything gets down to a calculated risk."

"But we don't really have a choice, do we," she said as statement, not as question.

Leachman shook his head from side to side. "Dr. Cooley'll be by tonight to talk with you. You make your decision and tell him."

A few doors down was a teen-age Italian boy, who seemingly had been making a textbook recovery from his heart surgery but whose prosperous-looking father was now distraught over a peculiar-looking patch of something that had appeared on the back of his son's head. Almost weeping, he implored Leachman with gesture, in a mixture of Italian and English, to inspect the suspicious growth. Leachman seemed puzzled and took the boy's head in his hands. He had to bite his lips to keep from laughing. "How do you say, 'Head and Shoulders' in Italian?" he said to the nurse. "The kid's got a big patch of dandruff. All he needs is a shampoo."

A Venezuelan baby, chubby, with huge dark solemn eyes, toddled down the hall, waving at the older children riding up and about the corridor in wheelchairs. Kids bounce back fast and they are encouraged to get out of their beds and play, even if it means hide-and-go-seek in the nursing station or bumper cars in the foyer. Leachman picked up the baby and laughed with him. "Cooley did a low-risk palliative procedure last week. Mario here is the classic blue baby, he has Tetralogy of Fallot, which is four major heart defects. He'll have to come back for more surgery in a few years."

Adult patients were also in Texas Children's, stashed there temporarily until the additions to St. Luke's were finished. Leachman's first stop was to see a cheerful, thirtyish fellow who had sailed through his surgery, but whose teeth had all fallen out afterward in adverse reaction to a drug. It was one of those weird side effects that could not be anticipated and that plague doctors.

"Did you eat your breakfast this morning?" asked Leachman.

"All except a hard piece of toast I couldn't gum to death."

"Well, at least you can honestly say, 'Look, Ma, no cavities.'"

"Dr. Leachman, do you know if Blue Cross pays to put a fellow's teeth back in?"

"Sure don't. I'll look into it, though."

It was almost noon, but Leachman was not half done with rounds. Cooley and DeBakey would have seen ten times this number of patients within the two hours that Leachman had prowled the wards. But patients sit in their beds all day long waiting for the big moment of the doctor's appearance, and when one like Leachman strolls in—one who does not seem in a rush to get out—the patient takes advantage of it.

"You've got heart palpitations, all right," said Leachman to an elderly, heavy woman. "But we don't think you need surgery just now. We'll treat it medically for a while and watch it."

The woman cut in hurriedly. "But I'm not too old for surgery, am I?"

"How many years you owning up to?"

"Sixty-nine."

"You may be too *young* for surgery."

"Oh God, oh merciful sweet Jesus, I'm so glad. Doctors used to discriminate against older people. .. . . Well, if surgery is ever indicated, I certainly want it. I want to live as long as, I can. . . . That's not being selfish, is it?"

Leachman shook his head in agreement. "I think every patient should have the medical facts and apply them to himself and then make his own decision about surgery. But you can go on home now and stay in touch."

The woman lifted her arm. There was a Band-Aid at the crook of the elbow where the catheterization probe had been injected. Two stitches were there to close the small incision. "I'll take these out myself at home," she said.

"Can't do that," said Leachman. "Against union rules. Somebody'll be around later today to take them out." He patted her arm and made to leave.

Leachman went off to search for his cigar; he had momentarily forgotten where he laid it down. "Is it true what she said?" I asked, "that they used to discriminate against older people?"

He nodded. "Still do, as a matter of fact. A lot of surgeons wouldn't touch a woman that old. We didn't used to do many, but we're a little more confident and knowledgeable now. Some of our confreres, however, are continually concerned about their batting averages."

The last patient of the morning was Harold Carstairs of Illinois. He had checked in the night before and this was Leachman's first visit. Carstairs already had been worked up by the cardiology and surgical divisions. They had confirmed with their stethoscopes what the hometown doctor had suspected—grave heart disease, a whopping hole in the heart called a ventricular septal defect. The hole had been there for years, possibly since Carstairs' birth 49 years ago, and the heart had been forced to beat harder than it should have, enlarging it as surely as the muscle on a man's arm enlarges when he picks up heavy crates every day.

"Does your heart bother *you*," asked Leachman as an introduction, "or does it just bother your doctors?"

"I read the obituaries every night to make sure I'm still alive," answered Carstairs in a quiet little voice. He was a short, average-looking man with thinning hair well oiled and combed back behind his ears. There was the same sadness about him that had enveloped Pamela Kroger in Children's two hours earlier.

"Did you get any breakfast?"

"Not much."

"Well, we try to make you suffer as much as possible and at the same time cut down on hospital expense."

"You think Dr. Cooley's going to operate on me?"

"We're not at that plateau just yet." Leachman spoke carefully. The man's heart was as gross and flabby as an overripe pumpkin. It could stop and give out during surgery or after surgery or —for that matter—while Leachman was talking to him. "We're going to do this catheterization on you this afternoon, and if it shows what your doctor back home thinks it will show, then we'll come back and talk to you some more."

Carstairs' eyes had been clear during Leachman's earlier remarks, but suddenly they began to cloud. He cleared his throat and spoke hesitantly in a voice that was difficult to hear. "I wanted to say . . . it's just that I'm ready. . . ."

Leachman smiled. He slapped him gently on the leg. He walked outside and hurried back to cardiology. "That's one sick boy," he murmured. "I wonder how they live long enough to get here."

In Leachman's absence, little had improved in the cardiology lab. There were patients still waiting for catheterizations, phones were still ringing, the Spanish voices were still caught up in urgent debate over another EKG. I would learn in the months to come that chaos often defeated order in the burdened chambers of Cooley's heart institute. The surgeon had thrown enormous pressure onto the hospitals: cases flowed out of his operating rooms and jammed the Recovery Room and Intensive Care and the wards and the waiting rooms. Everything from x-ray to the snack bar felt the weight of the numbers and not until the seven new floors of the Texas Heart Institute were open would there be abatement. Everyone complained, everyone said they were overworked, but somehow people got operated on and most of them got well. An anesthesiologist would tell me, "In Houston, success means numbers. First and Most. If a patient wants tender, loving care, he's not going to get it from Denton Cooley or Mike DeBakey."

Dr. Leachman slipped into his cubbyhole office and sat down gratefully. "Surgery, you see," he began immediately, starting a new topic but launching into it as if he had been lecturing on it all morning, "is a tremendous injury, a major insult. Surgery is like . . . like getting hit by a car! The critical period is not only when the patient is on the operating table, it is the 24 hours, the 48 hours afterward. Will the heart stand the new circulation process? Will the lungs take the new pressure? Sometimes the surgeon eliminates the mechanical defect that he is hired to do, but if the heart is so sick that it cannot accommodate the repair, if it cannot assume the new work, then the patient will die. But he will die in the recovery room or in his own room or at home, and the surgeon has long since washed his hands of it."

One of the South American cardiology fellows appeared abruptly with a catheterization report and an EKG trailing on the floor. He said it strongly suggested the patient in question would be a good candidate for the coronary artery bypass—the operation Ted Diethrich had done on Arthur Bingham, the procedure which was the number one topic in the heart surgery business. One of the few it had not excited—yet—was Denton Cooley who, hospital gossip had it, thoroughly disliked the meticulous, lengthy procedure. Gossip in a hospital is no more reliable than gossip anywhere else, only there is more of it. One reason is the insularity of medicine; the nature of medical work is that it tends to shut out the world beyond, locking both patients and personnel within. (A few months later, St. Luke's would be boarded up for a threatened hurricane. With doors and windows covered, the hospital seemed physically what it had always been spiritually—a womb.) One of the gossips, a general surgeon, had commented that Cooley simply could not afford the time required for the new operation. "Denton's got himself in a bind; he's got to operate eight, ten times a day to bring in the revenue for his various projects. If he does the coronary properly, it'd mean cutting his list in half."

Leachman shot that notion down.

"It takes a lot of time, true," he said, "but there are other reasons. I'm not yet sold on whether the operation does anything but cut down anginal pain. It's too early to tell if it does anything for longevity, because the surgeons have only been doing them in big numbers for a year or so."

He stopped and picked up the reports the younger doctor had left on his desk. "Take this fellow. . . . He's, let me see, he's 47 years old, one previous heart attack, he's probably building up to another. He's got bad anginal pain. So what we're dealing with here are two main problems: one, suffering from pain, and two, suffering from the threat of death. This patient has coronary artery disease, a disease that you and me and every single one of us is going to get sooner or later if we don't die from car wrecks or gun shot or air pollution. We might even say that aging is nothing more than the process which occurs in our arteries. But there are other facts that can bring on this condition besides age—diabetes, hypertension, the hereditary factor, civilization as a whole. You can almost measure a country's progress when its statistics on heart deaths start to go up. I went to Venezuela years ago and there were very few heart cases; their babies were dying of diarrhea and the adults of tuberculosis. Now Venezuela is either an emerging or a developing nation and its people are dropping dead from heart attacks. And they're almost proud of it! Like the Russians were when they started reporting their coronary statistics at world meetings.

"So, how do we go about dealing with massive disease? We can try to *prevent* it in the first place by proper diet, activities, drugs, but *prevent* is a strong word. What we are really doing is stalling if off longer. If we ever got to the point where we could prevent atherosclerosis, we'd have people living to be 150, 200 years old. That would almost be an immoral act on the doctors' part. We could be guilty of the ultimate population explosion. And if the medical profession ever achieves that goal, then the politicians are going to move in fast and restrict the kind of people we will be allowed to keep alive. Here we have the Mudd Family, for example, five documented generations of incest, murder, rape, and thieving. How much of our food and living space shall we allow them to use? I can see the catchy headline now, 'We've Got Too Many People: Who's Going to Go?' "

"But," I asked, "wouldn't birth control at the start avoid this?"

"Nope. The desirable people of our society are already restricting their families; the undesirables won't and never will. But we're digressing. Maybe what we should do to get at heart disease is to study the population—take the families with no diabetes or coronary artery disease, the families with 'good genes,' and breed them with the ones who are most liable to die of heart attacks. This would be one way to attack coronary disease—breeding control."

Leachman was out of cigars so he bummed a cigarette. Next to a minister who drinks, there is nothing more comforting to a sinner than a doctor who smokes. "Now, this super-duper new operation, this venous bypass. Granted, it is the first operation that seems relatively logical. But it is nothing more, so far, than a palliative procedure at best—and there are many other ways to reduce the pain from angina. We can always cut the nerves leading to a guy's heart and he won't feel a thing. Not even the heart attack that finally kills him."

Denton Cooley finished his eighth case of the day at 5:35 and lightly placed a gauze sponge into the incision of the heart, his unspoken signal that the first assistant was to take over and close.

Neither Cooley nor DeBakey has the time to make the initial incision
or the final sewing up. This is fairly common practice among important surgeons; were they to do the case from "skin to skin" it
would take an average of three to four hours. (At a cocktail party
in New York several months after my return from Houston, I met
a businessman from Long Island who told me of his surgery by De-
Bakey. He was so overwhelmed by his good health that he stripped
off his coat, unbuttoned his shirt, and displayed a well-healed scar,
stretching from Adam's apple to navel. "Professor DeBakey did
this," he said, as if showing off a first folio Shakespeare. I congratulated him on his recovery and decided against spoiling his notion of
authorship.)

Rounds would commence as soon as Cooley went out and told the
families what had happened to their loved ones in surgery that day,
a job he executed with as much speed and dispatch as the operations
themselves. He strode quickly down the hall to a crowded waiting
room outside Leachman's lab where he pulled out a small filing card
with names written on it. Fifty people stopped talking and someone
shut off the television set.

"Mrs. Brown?" Mrs. Brown hurried up, pale, haggard. "Your husband's fine; we put in a new aortic valve in his heart. He's just going
to recovery now and you can go in and see him at seven. . . ."

"Mrs. Green?" Mrs. Green was lurking nearby, waiting, fearing
her turn. She had an autograph book in her hand but first she would
learn of Mr. Green. "He's fine, just fine. We put in a Dacron graft
right where we told him we would. . . . You can see him in the
recovery room at seven."

"Mr. Jones?" Mr. Jones was helped to his feet by two grown
daughters, he being an aged, wrinkled man who had been mentally
standing beside his wife's grave all day. "Your wife is fine. She took
the surgery very well. You can see her in the recovery room at
seven."

They all had questions, but Cooley was gone, vanishing around
the corner and on his way back to surgery. Silent, elegant, giant
steps on rubber-cushioned soles. How could the relatives know that
he rarely spoke, even to the patients? He was in and out of rooms
at times without uttering a syllable, sometimes a nod, other times only
a touch at the foot of the bed where the strip of tape bears the name of

the patient and the disease and his name. The only time he was at total ease was in his operating rooms, where he was among his friends, where the only strangers were those on his table and by the time he saw them they had become abstract figures in the medical landscape, openings in green drapes. "He's done 69 pumps in the last nine days!" exclaimed a surgical fellow named John Zaorski as he waited for Cooley to change from greens to street dress. "Pumps" are open-heart cases in which the oxygenating machine is used. "I spent a year at the leading hospital in New Jersey and we did 35 pumps the whole twelve months. The man is incredible. The man is absolutely a magician."

The man is also obsessed. He operates beyond fatigue, beyond endurance. He once broke two ribs water skiing, had them bound, and attended surgery the next day. A horse kicked him at his ranch and broke his leg; he ordered a cylinder cast put on it and hobbled to the table where he did a full schedule. In pain from a hernia, he operated an entire day, then lay down on his own table and permitted his associate, Grady Hallman, to repair it. Within two days he was operating again, and in his haste, he had torn his stitches. His back went out on a golf course and he could not straighten up; an ambulance picked him up like a jack knife. But he did not miss a day. In recent weeks he had suffered from a kidney stone and thrombosed hemorrhoids, two conditions that can make a strong man cry out, but he would not stop working.

"Denton would rather operate than fuck," said a longtime friend and associate. "And I've never seen him give less than his best, even when we've been called back to the hospital from a party at midnight and we both had to chew gum before we could go into the operating room."

Another friend from medical-school years has long since stopped trying to fathom the man. "I can understand why someone would drive himself that way when he is young and trying to make his name, his reputation," said the friend. "But Denton was honored for his one-thousandth open heart at least seven years ago. Who can approach that? Life is a competition for him; in our generation, the people who were looked up to were the competitors."

He is not an approachable man. He would seem to feel that the public needs to know but two marks of his heroism: he is handsome, he is skilled. Perhaps a third. He has done the most. He does not even permit himself the changes of mood of other surgeons. Changes can betray an image, and Cooley has carefully constructed his. DeBakey shouts; another Houston surgeon has been known to fall to his knees and beat his gloved fists against the operating-room floor in despair; still another throws up his hands and cries, "Won't somebody *please* help me?" Cooley grows impatient, and impatience breeds anger, but his anger is masked behind a muttered sarcasm or, worse, half an hour of complete silence. The friend from medical school remarked: "Even at sixteen he was an enigma to all of us. He had an aura about him. He was one of those golden boys—now a man—whom you don't feel quite at ease around. It is almost as if you are afraid you will make a mistake. I feel insecure; I feel uncomfortable in his presence and I am supposed to be his oldest friend."

Cooley had a tiny office, perhaps four feet wide by six feet long, on an elevated platform with windows overlooking Operating Room 1 but two feet below, and here he had gone to change. He drew on dark trousers, a lemon shirt with a monogram on the pocket, a widely knotted tie. DeBakey charges about his hospital in surgical scrub with occasional flecks of blood on his uniform. Cooley glides through his, tailored, immaculate, his lab coat pristine white.

Trailed by his dozen surgical fellows, all from foreign countries except for John Zaorski, Cooley stopped in the jammed, turbulent Recovery Room and touched the foot of the bed of a young Ceylonese girl. "This is a gratuitous operation," he said, and moved on. A surgeon in Ceylon had attempted to correct her Tetralogy of Fallot, had botched it, and had sent her to Houston. She would fly home, radiant, in two weeks.

"Gratuitous," as I use the word, has more than one meaning; I asked Cooley which he was using. "Free. Gratis," Cooley said. "And so is he." He pointed to a painfully thin, elongated Asian-looking patient thrashing about in his bed, just coming around from anesthesia. One of the fellows murmured that he was Pakistani. He had an atrial septal defect, which Cooley had just repaired.

The Pakistani had flown to Houston without an appointment and had talked a cab driver into taking him to Cooley's home in the exclusive River Oaks section of Houston. There he had presented himself for treatment; the maid sent him to the hospital, where Cooley performed the surgery. Ten days later he was complaining loudly that the hospital bill was outrageous and he should receive a "student discount."

Little Pamela Kroger had been yelling at doctors and nurses all day, but when Cooley walked into her room smiling, she hushed. Even at four, she had respect for his celebrity. "Hello, honey," he said, able to press his stethoscope against her heart and listen to the hissing irregularities without interruptions. He beckoned for Mrs. Kroger to follow him outside. She had talked to several doctors during the day and she well understood her option: take the child home and wait for her heart to stop, or agree to the nightmare of a man plunging his hands into the child's heart, in a room where she, the mother, could not go.

"I think we can fix her up," Cooley began. "But. . . ."

"I know," she said. She had been wrestling over what she would say at this moment, and now it was time, and she was nearly mute.

Cooley helped her. "If she was my little girl, I'd have it done. I wouldn't like it, but I'd agree to it. I just want you to know there is a risk, though."

Mrs. Kroger stood silent for several moments, not aware that Cooley was anxious to be about his rounds. Finally she nodded her consent, began to cry, ashamed at breaking down in front of this man. She rushed back into her daughter's room, a hand thrown across her face to conceal the tears from the child.

Outside another room, Cooley told Harold Carstairs' wife, "This is high-risk surgery. The hole in his heart has been there for a long time, possibly since birth. We can repair that—that's not the problem. It's the three or four days later that we worry about."

"What are the odds?" she asked. Patients and relatives always like to know the odds, as if there was a tote board for all lesions.

Cooley pursed his lips and pulled a figure at random. "About eight to five," he said and walked away. He muttered to John Russell, his resident, "I hate to make book in front of the patients' wives."

One of the Iranian fellows caught Zaorski's sleeve. "What did he say?" Zaorski explained what odds were and what a bookie was. "He talks so fast and so quiet I can't understand him," said the Iranian.

A voluptuous Eurasian mother wearing a mini skirt hesitantly walked up to Cooley, and in struggling English, said, "For you," shoving a carefully wrapped package into his hands. Cooley thanked her and opened it, discovering a heavy, quite hideous statue of an ancient anonymous doctor or professor. Later, on the floor below, he looked at it again, grimaced, and said, as he handed it to an intern, "I guess I could always put trifocals on it and call it St. Michael."

"What did he say?" asked one of the foreign doctors.

Zaorski gestured with his head toward Methodist.

On the eve of open-heart surgery, a man lies unfed in his bed and waits for the Nembutal to darken the strange walls. Harold Carstairs was bewildered. A simple man who had worked hard all of his life, he could not understand why he had been chosen to joust with death at the age of 49. He had pitched hay on a farm until he was 21 and thought himself to be a robust youth until the Army rejected him in 1946 because of a heart murmur. A heart murmur! Perhaps he had been born with it, perhaps it had come from an unknown attack of rheumatic fever. It so frightened him that he buried all thoughts of it, and when it threatened him he ran away from it, as a man runs from a criminal past. "A person has to work," he said. "I got a job on a towboat picking up 85-pound rachets and carrying them around. I worked on the Illinois Central Railroad for ten years and I never once took the physical. I always figured out a way to avoid it. I thought if they heard my heart they would fire me."

Six years before, a doctor told him to have his heart examined by a specialist. "But he didn't press me about it, so I didn't do it." Not until six months before this Houston night had enough apprehension set in for him to find a heart doctor. He had begun to cough and could not drink enough syrup to make it stop. He felt generally run down and had begun, as he discreetly put it, "to lose my desire."

Now his apprehension had turned to fright. He clutched his wife's hand. "I've got so much back home," he said. "I've got this wonderful family, the best a man ever had. . . ." "I never did anything bad to anybody. . . ." His tears were splashing down his face and, as men do when there is nothing else, he turned to his faith. "I had a vision last night. I saw Dr. Cooley walk in with his young doctors and I swore it was Jesus Christ and his Disciples."

Super-Jesus!

CHAPTER

6

Dr. Jerry Strong bent over Pamela and blotted her perspiring face. She had been sedated in her room, but the tranquilizers were beginning to wear off as she lay on the stretcher outside Operating Room 1. She was whimpering slightly. Strong said softly, "It's all right, honey, it's all right. We're going to put you to sleep and fix you up in just a minute." He went into the coffee room and said to no one in particular, "Pulmonary pressure like that kid's is a bomb with a 72-hour fuse."

Slender, witty, caustic, and a highly skilled anesthesiologist, Strong reigned as raconteur of the coffee room, the crowded lounge just inside the swinging doors that led to surgery. There were no windows in the lounge and the furniture was cheap, cracking tan plastic; the ashtrays were overflowing, the magazines were out of date. But it served as unofficial headquarters for Cooley's domain. Throughout the day and half the night it was crowded with surgeons resting before, after, or sometimes during their cases, nurses grabbing a cigarette, medical students cramming or listening to their elders talk of patients and politics. The main attraction was the free hot coffee, and, on days that the drug detail men came around, blueberry cupcakes or oatmeal cookies with a foul-tasting orange ribbon on top. Cooley's fellows drifted in after each case to dictate surgical reports, and they assembled there each afternoon to discuss the day's work and await his appearance for rounds.

There was an aura about the two heart teams at the two hospitals which went beyond the marked physical differences in space and resources. (A Cooley staff doctor had complained during the transplant year that he was a man using a $2\frac{1}{2}$-horsepower lawn-mower engine while DeBakey's people, in their splendiforous center, had a 450-horsepower Cadillac.) Each surgeon dominated his hospital and each used power in his own fashion, but a nurse at St. Luke's did not even bother to lower her voice in the coffee room when she announced that she did not enjoy scrubbing for Cooley. "I've had Dr. Wonderful and his God Squad," she said. "I'll take orthopedics."

Two visiting doctors were in the coffee room with name tags stuck on their scrubs indicating they were from out of state. They had arrived early to watch Pamela's surgery. They took coffee from the big urn and wandered out to look at the blackboard in the foyer, with the first twelve spaces usually occupied by Cooley cases. A student who had been talking with them remarked on the large number of physicians continually pouring through Houston and crowding Cooley's—and DeBakey's—tables.

"We get all the VIP's down here," said Dr. Jerry Strong, as he tied on his throwaway sterile mask. "Let's face it; this *is* the Big Top."

At 7:45 A.M., Dr. Domingo Liotta, an Argentine-born surgeon and researcher sliced open Pamela's emaciated chest. Shortly after 8 A.M., when her ribs were parted and the enlarged heart exposed, Cooley entered the room and, while a nurse dressed him in his sterile gown, asked someone to turn the radio up a little. He says he is not conscious of the music, even though he often whistles or hums along with it, but it is part of his room, as are the cartoons, the occasional nude picture, the inspirational posters that decorate the sterile walls where he spends most of his life with these sayings:

"Ideas won't keep—something must be done about them."

"Yesterday is gone, tomorrow may never come, now is the appointed hour."

"The more you help another, the more you help yourself."

And, dominating all, a long quotation from Theodore Roosevelt:

"The credit belongs to the man who is actually in the arena, whose face is marred by dust and sweat and blood . . . who knows the great enthusiasms, the great devotions and who spends himself in a worthy cause . . . who at the end at best knows the triumph of high achievement and at worse fails while daring greatly, so that his place will never be with those cold and timid souls who know neither victory nor defeat."

Always it is the same. Always there is the one suspended moment when he looks down through the gold Italian half-spectacles taped lightly to his blond, graying sideburns, seeing for the first time the troubled heart beating beneath him. ("Can you remember the first heart you ever saw?" I once asked him. He thought for a moment and finally shook his head. "There've been too many," he answered. I had asked the same question of DeBakey, only he remembered. He said, in fact, he could never forget it. It was in the early 1930s, in the emergency room of Charity Hospital in New Orleans; he had looked down through the rib cage and seen a tiny pulsing pink part of a heart that had been pierced with a knife in a brawl.)

With a slight shift of his shoulder, Cooley was off, hands boldly slipping into the once forbidden chamber, carpentering a new system of circulation within Pamela's heart. "Some surgeons piddle," a doctor remarked after watching Cooley operate. "Some surgeons fool around and step back from the table and play with the sucking machine and poke around inside the patient. But not him. He doesn't waste a breath, not a gesture. He knows exactly where he is going because he has been there before."

Only twice during the delicate procedure—how simple it looked! —did he speak. Once was in reply to the visiting doctor who asked how often Pamela's disease—transposition of the great vessels—was encountered. "We used to think it was rare," he said, "but it is now known to be one of the most common congenital defects. The trouble is, so many kids die when they are a few weeks old." The second was when he glanced behind him through the glass walls into Room 2, where the next case was being prepared. "What's that?" he asked. A nurse went to check the schedule sheet posted by the scrub basin. "The vsp," she said, giving the abbreviation for ventricular septal defect.

That's not a "what." That's not a vsp. That is a human male, one Harold Carstairs from Illinois. Next to his birth, next to his death, this is the biggest moment of his life. Must he be anonymous? Had Cooley connected the cavity before him with the child Pamela he saw yesterday for thirty seconds or the mother he saw for forty? Was it possible to hold so many hearts in his hands and *know* them?

"Denton Cooley," said a friend who stood once and watched him through the glass, "is the greatest doctor in the world—from here down." He made a slashing gesture, a line of demarcation across the wrists.

It was gray and misty with thunder dancing about the city, a condition that seemed compatible with the mood of Marsha Kroger as she waited news of Pamela. Beside her was her divorced husband Gerald, Pamela's father, a chunky, gentle man with a crew cut and a soft north-Louisiana drawl that welded words together. He had both a book of philosophy and *Dr. Zhivago* on his lap, but every time footsteps approached, his eyes shot up from the page. Certain people become familiar during the waiting—nurses, orderlies pushing carts, but when a new figure appears, the families are swept by panic. Is the message coming?

"A month after Pamela was born, she turned a bluish color," recalled Mrs. Kroger. She was a slim woman with an air of efficiency about her. "A strange duskiness set in. Her eyes had always troubled me, a child that sick has haunting eyes. We sat there with our Dr. Spock, trying to be good parents. Our pediatrician didn't even recognize heart problems. He kept saying she wasn't feeding properly.

"The thing that began to frighten me was the memory of my twin sisters who died of heart defects a few weeks after they were born. And my grandmother had twin sons, uncles I never knew, who had died of what they called 'malnutrition' then, but which was probably heart disease. I felt I was carrying the bad seed and had passed it on to my daughter. . . . On the day Pamela sank into heart failure, our pediatrician finally decided we should rush her to Houston. Gerald couldn't get an ambulance. . . ."

Her ex-husband winced at the recollection. "There was a water festival going on at the lake and all the ambulances in Austin were out there hoping to pick up a drowning. . . ."

"He finally chartered a plane," said Mrs. Kroger, picking up the story. "They flew her to Houston and arrived at Texas Children's with sirens blaring. They did her first catheterization the day Charles Whitman was shooting people from the University of Texas tower. When we got the diagnosis, that the great vessels of the heart were transposed, Gerald fainted."

Gerald nodded, not embarrassed at the memory. "I was ready to accept one of the minor heart defects, a murmur, even a hole, because I knew Cooley could do them. But this sounded so staggering I thought we would surely lose her."

"When she got old enough," said Mrs. Kroger, lighting a new cigarette from the one she had not yet finished, "we told her about her condition. Sometimes she referred to her 'sick heart' with a cute look on her face, but she never used it as an excuse. Living with a heart baby was hell. You try to protect her, but you also try to let her lead a normal life. The other day she was on the monkey bars at the park and she froze—she got tired and pale and I could see her anguish."

Two hours and forty minutes after she had entered the operating room whimpering, time bomb Pamela was ready to leave, her heart reconstructed, her existence for the time dependent upon technology. Jerry Strong supervised her transfer from the table to the rolling stretcher. "Patients not infrequently arrest between here and there," he said, pointing down the hall toward Recovery. "So I think it's important to stay with them all the way." A tube was down her throat and its connection taped across her mouth for the ventilator that would breathe for her until the lungs rallied—if they could. During the transfer, Strong would squeeze the black oxygen bag to feed her with oxygen.

"What are you bringing us?" said one of the Recovery nurses as

Strong and an orderly delivered Pamela. "Transposition," said Strong. A place was made at the end of the room where the children are watched.

Dr. Liotta had come out between surgery and hovered as the nurses hooked up Pamela to the various monitoring machines and wrote her name on the strip of tape at the foot of her bed. Leachman was in Recovery checking on another patient and moved down to Pamela's bed. "She'll be all right if the cardiologist takes proper care of her," said Liotta.

Leachman watched the surgeon return to his quarters. "This is the surgeon's out, don't you see," he said. "He has committed this massive assault on the patient and now he passes the buck to me."

(Near midnight, Leachman was attending Pamela and he said, not wholly in jest, "Note what physician is still here and what famous surgeon went home hours ago.")

The general feeling was that Harold Carstairs had small chance of surviving. "I'll be surprised if he gets off the table," said one of the surgical fellows, looking at the x-rays that Gwen, the head operating room nurse, had slapped onto the illuminated viewer in the corner of Room 2. The heart was enormous, its shadowy shape almost as big as the chest itself. Strong glanced at it and shook his head, virtually a shudder. But there was no curtain of pessimism in the room, where a Muzak-type station had been switched to one that sent out hard rock, the room where Harold Carstairs was probably going to die. "In medical school," a cardiologist named Don Rochelle would tell me, "you start out by having enormous empathy for patients and their families. You get involved with all of them. But to work in the cardiovascular field, you have to develop almost a shield around you. When someone dies, they die. You can't crack up—caths go on, surgery goes on. There'll be twelve new patients in tomorrow."

Liotta was first-assisting all day, opening the chests, following Cooley on the sutures, finally closing. The job was passed around on a rotation basis to all twelve of the surgical fellows, plus Liotta, who spent most of his time up in the seventh-floor lab in research but who relished the rare opportunity to cut and sew. When Liotta exposed Carstairs' heart, Jerry Strong glanced at it and made an inverted whistle. "Jesus, would you look at that! It's one of the worst-looking hearts I've ever seen. Most of these cases die by the time they're 35. It's wall-to-wall heart!"

The huge heart was so flaccid and deteriorated that Cooley had to go at the ventricular septal defect through the tricuspid valve, roughly equivalent to entering a house by crawling under the basement door. During surgery, Jerry Strong pinched Carstairs' cheeks now and then, bringing a momentary cosmetic flush of pink to the pale skin. Anesthesiologists do this to see if blood is flowing to the patient's head.

"This is known as the George Lewis technique," Strong said.

"Is that a professor here?" asked one of the visiting doctors.

"He's a local undertaker."

One of the visitors, a short doctor unable to see the field, had navigated his way to the patient's head-end of the table and was standing on a large, shaky stool. Gwen eyed him nervously and finally asked him to get down, diplomatically finding him a better place. "Someday somebody is going to fall into the patient," she muttered.

"How old is this patient?" asked the short doctor from his new position.

Cooley shook his head. "Gwen?"

Gwen found the chart with the plastic identification card and discovered from it that Carstairs was 49.

The short doctor shook his head in disbelief, as well he might have.

Carstairs probably was born with the hole in his septum, that partition that separates the two ventricles (lower chambers) of his heart. This had caused the right ventricle to work furiously, pumping blood into the lungs, and at the same time fighting off pressure from the left ventricle. Blood that had returned from the lungs with oxygen had continually mixed with blood that was on its way to the lungs. The ventricular septal defect is the most common congenital heart defect and is almost routinely corrected by the heart surgeons —both Cooley and DeBakey had mortality rates under 10 percent, But Carstairs' heart was so gross and the tissue around the hole so worn and tired that it would take a large patch to cover it. Would the sutures even hold? Would any other surgeon have even attempted it?

Gwen handed, without being asked, a Dacron patch to Cooley, which he accepted and with his scissors trimmed down to a circular affair, larger than a quarter and smaller than a half-dollar. Deftly he sewed it into the septum, closing off the hole. He worked calmly, dispassionately. Disasters have happened—they happen in any surgery—but none has ever broken his calm. A clamp can slip off an aorta and blood can erupt to the ceiling like a geyser. Cooley sews through the blood. Once an assisting surgeon was opening the chest with an electric saw and he cut too far, slicing into the heart. He cried out in horror. Cooley hurried into the room, quietly sewed up the unintended wound, and turned to the defect for which he had been engaged.

When he was done with Carstairs' patch Cooley said, almost in a whisper, "Let's see what happens." Carstairs was taken off the pump and the life-sustaining responsibility given back to his own system. The heart fibrillated slightly, enough to cause Cooley to put him back on the pump for another few moments. A jolt of electricity started up the heart the second time. It beat regularly and normally.

Jerry Strong raised his eyebrows as a compliment to Cooley's surgery, also indicating that there was considerable road to travel before the reconstruction could be considered successful.

Three hours after Pamela's surgery, her blood pressure was up to 82/50, a good sign. She was trembling, moving her arms about, and fighting the mouthpiece as the anesthesia began to slip from her system.

After six more operations, Cooley finished at 5 P.M., made brief rounds, visiting those patients whom John Russell had scheduled for the next day. A mother whose child was recovering nicely asked if he would pose for a photograph. Not only would he, he swooped up the child, instructed the woman to move across the room with her back to the afternoon sun, and held still for one Polaroid and two 35mm slides. A second woman watching expressed disappointment that she had not brought her camera. Did Cooley have any pictures of himself? His office would give her one. Cooley hands out handsome line drawings from a Karsh portrait. DeBakey has a stack of glossies he autographs and distributes to those who ask. It occurred to me that there are two professions where the participant stands directly under a spotlight—acting and surgery—while doing their principal work.

I had an appointment to eat dinner at a Mexican restaurant with two medical student friends, and as I dressed, another student was combing his hair in the locker room. He had been working in Cooley's surgery that day, doing the scut work of holding retractors until the fingers ache and pinpoints of pain invade them.

"Some day," I said. "Eight cases."

"That's too many," said the student. "Personally I think the surgeon should do fewer cases and have more rapport with the patient. Some surgeons actually work up the patient preoperatively, do the operation, and stay with him until he is out of danger."

But who could do as many sophisticated cases as Cooley can do? "Shouldn't his skill be used on as many patients as possible?"

The student shook his head. He had long sideburns and the beginnings of a mustache. Jerry Strong had commented that very day how hip the medical students were starting to look. "Wait till the AMA gets ahold of them," Strong had said.

"There might be other Cooleys around if somebody gave them the chance," the youth said. "But of course I'm still a student, and I'm still idealistic."

Medical students know of all the places where dinner is cheap and filling. This being Wednesday it was half-price night at a Mexican restaurant where for 99 cents one got a taco, a combination plate of enchiladas, beans, rice, tamales, a basket full of toasted tortillas, and heartburn (a misnomer, it should be called esophagus burn, because the heart is not involved). Jerry Naifeh and Bob Viles, both second-year students and aspiring surgeons—in their classes, when a theoretical case would be presented and the instructor would ask for possible medical solutions, Jerry and Bob would usually cry, "Cut! Cut!"—were talking about DeBakey's announced scheme to reduce the number of years a doctor must spend in medical school and residency before he can begin practicing. As it then stood, a heart surgeon had to spend thirteen or fourteen years after he finished college, making him almost 35 by the time he had fulfilled his military obligations. The training period was four years in medical school, one year in internship, four years in a residency, three years in a surgical specialty, and one year as a fellow.

DeBakey had recently proposed cutting one year out of medical school—"the second's a waste of time, anyway," said Jerry—and shortening the residency from four years to three. In a nation critically short of doctors, it seemed a valid idea. Most doctors think they are over-trained anyway.

"The Professor's always looking out for the students," said Jerry. "He's almost a God to us."

It was not always thus. Less than a handful of years ago DeBakey was so caught up in his myriad duties that students complained they never saw him or had access to him. At the annual senior dinner, the class voted DeBakey their "Chicken" award, given by graduating students to the faculty member who had contributed *least* to their medical education. Stung, DeBakey instituted a series of Saturday-morning breakfasts at which all seniors were invited for free bacon and eggs and an ask-me-anything hour.

Jerry suggested that DeBakey erupts at people in his operating room to weed out those emotionally unfit to become surgeons. "He really psyches you out if you let him," said Jerry. "You make mistakes, you forget everything when he goes on a rampage. There was this woman resident who really got it. He used to scream at her, 'No, deah, no! You'll never learn! You're psychologically defeated!'" (The woman is now a successful Houston surgeon.)

Hans Paessler joined us, weary after three afternoon cases with Ted Diethrich and an hour in the lab inducing heart attacks in pigs. Hans looked like a ski instructor with wide shoulders and strong arms. He was spending his year in Houston not only observing De-Bakey and Diethrich but wheeling his yellow Fiat convertible about the southwestern part of the city in heavy pursuit of beautiful and preferably rich girls. "I have a date this weekend with a former Miss Playmate," said Hans. "She works at the Shamrock Hilton as a hostess."

"As a *what?*" said Jerry.

"She greets visiting dignitaries," said Hans. "She is . . . she has."

Hans was searching in vain for English dimensional terminology. He settled for extending his hands a considerable distance in front of his chest.

"Medicine is business in Houston," Hans said, taking a sip of Lone Star beer and frowning, mentally comparing it with the brew of Munich. "The patient is the customer. I've never seen a place like this. Doctors are so nice to each other! The reason is they worry constantly about getting referrals. I asked a cardiologist the other day why he was always smiling, always so polite to everybody, and he said, 'Because you never can tell who's going to give me a referral some day.' "

In his country, Hans said, surgeons do not operate on the very elderly. "We send an 85-year-old woman with an aneurysm back to her cabbage patch and let her live out her life. Here, DeBakey will operate on her. It's incredible!"

I drove back quickly to St. Luke's, where I wanted to follow the progress of Pamela and Carstairs through the most critical night of their lives. John Zaorski was on night duty, looking after all of Cooley's patients. Zaorski, a stocky, crew-cut reserve major in the Air Force and a former sugeon with the military in Korea, was on the last leg of his medical education. At 35, he was anxious to get into private practice. The nursing staff considered him one of the best of the fellows—"They like me because at least I speak English," said John, who spoke in a rat-a-tat Joisey accent. He was coming out of a woman's room on Three South when I found him. "That's an interesting lady, you should talk to her," he said. "She's a Jehovah's Witness." The patient inside was Mrs. Grieg from Colorado, who had survived open-heart surgery without blood transfusion.

Cooley is one of the few surgeons in the world who will attempt surgery on Witnesses, having vowed to observe their prohibition against accepting blood. He has done some 100 cases, using only saline solution to replenish body fluids, and his mortality rate is about the same, in some series slightly lower, than with non-Witness patients. The feat is astonishing, considering that almost every surgery, even minor surgery, requires blood, if not during the actual operation, then certainly in the postoperative period.

The ban on blood for Witnesses is strictly observed; there is no cheating in Recovery when a pressure nose dives and the obvious treatment would be "give blood." Dr. Grady Hallman once noticed an order for blood written on a Witness chart and he quickly found the charge nurse and demanded an explanation. The nurse said that there had been an error, which had been caught, and that the blood had not been administered, only ordered.

Mrs. Grieg was a retired hairdresser, a neat, thin, prim woman, nine days postoperative. Her heart was tolerating the new plastic mitral valve that Cooley had put in. She was reading her Bible and she found a verse from Leviticus that is the foundation of their belief.

" 'Ye shall not eat blood. . . .' We interpret that as meaning that we cannot *use* blood, either. . . . 'It shall be poured out onto the ground.' " A bony, liver-spotted finger flew across the pages into the New Testament. "And St. Paul told us, right here, 'Ye shall abstain from blood.' Both the Old and the New Testament support our faith."

"Are there many dissenters to this principle within your sect?"

"Our organization has no splits. There are no rebels. We know only that it takes courage and we accept the risk. We believe that this is what God wants us to do, else he would not have given it to us in His Word. We cannot violate His Scriptures. When I entered the hospital, I signed a paper stating that, if I got anemia or postoperative complications, I would not hold the hospital or Dr. Cooley responsible. We think God is with us, He is in this room, He is listening to this conversation. We will remain alive only as long as He has need for us here."

Mrs. Grieg left the hospital the next day, looking serene and handing me some pamphlets to study.

Shortly after 10 P.M., Carstairs' potassium level dropped sharply, causing concern to Shirley Fife, the efficient Recovery Room nurse who was working a double shift, already having put in eight daytime hours in Leachman's cath lab. She took Carstairs' chart and hurried into the coffee room, where Zaorski was slumped for a few minutes rest. There had been few problems this night and on his last tour of the hospital, the nursing stations reported that everyone was either resting well, or better still, not complaining.

"This can be dangerous," Zaorski said, scanning the chart. "The danger is that the patient can go into arrhythmia, irregular heart beats; they can kill you. His potassium level is, let's see, 2.9. Normal is an even four. Potassium's an electrolyte, one of the chemical agents that controls the heart beat. Cooley foresaw this, because he hooked up Carstairs with pacemaker wires in case we needed to slap one on and speed up his beat."

Zaorski ordered potassium to be injected into Carstairs' intravenous tube and no sooner had he returned to his coffee than did Shirley hurry in, this time with Pamela's chart in hand. The child's potassium level also had plunged. "Give her some, too, as long as you're at it," said Zaorski.

In the hours after heart surgery, six danger signs watched for are:

1. Tamponade—bleeding around the heart. This can precipitate a fatal drop in blood pressure and must be corrected by emergency surgery. "This is usually the only thing we'd call Cooley for at home," said Zaorski. "This or a death."

2. Lung malfunction. The lungs can develop resistance to the new pressure system created by revised blood circulation within the heart.

3. Heart block. When the surgeon sews a patch into the heart, such as Carstairs' VSD repair, he must avoid hitting a vital clump of nerves called the Bundle of His. If a single suture is placed one millimeter over and into this clump, it can destroy the heart's natural pacing system and the patient must be hooked up to a pacemaker.

4. Low urine output, indicative that the kidneys are not being well nourished with blood pumped from the heart.

5. Arrhythmias.

6. Bleeding around the graft.

Shirley hauled Zaorski back into Recovery for the third time in less than half an hour. Pamela's intravenous tube had come out. "She probably pulled it out, she's been squirming and fighting everything," Shirley said. Zaorski sighed and tried for ten minutes to work an intravenous needle into Pamela's veins, but the child had been catheterized so often that her veins had thrombosed; they simply would not accept another needle.

"Gimme a cutdown," said Zaorski, requesting a sterile pack with instruments for cutting into the foot and finding a vein to hook up the intravenous.

The charge nurse, busy down the line turning a patient, called back, "You've got to get her parents' permission."

"For a cutdown?" Zaorski's voice was incredulous. A "cutdown" has long been a procedure of most routine nature.

"It's considered minor surgery now, and the hospital requires you to get the parents' signatures."

"Well, for Christ's sake that's a new one on me. What do you recommend? It's past midnight, visiting hours in most hospitals are over. You have any idea what motel I go to to find her parents? Or what their names are?"

The charge nurse shook her head. Zaorski asked me to scout the Texas Children's surgical waiting room; he, in the meantime, would look through St. Luke's lobby. I ran down the hall and into the dark foyer. An elderly man in cowboy boots was sleeping on a cot he had brought; he sat up with a startled look on his battered face. A woman trying to stretch across two folding chairs stood up quickly and searched for her eyeglasses. Neither belonged to Pamela. I apologized and raced back to Recovery. Zaorski had drawn a blank as well.

"The rule is," the nurse said, "that if the parents cannot be found and if the surgeon considers the procedure necessary, then he can go ahead."

Zaorski nodded. She could have saved us both a foot race.

"You just go ahead and start," said the nurse. "I'll phone around and try to find her parents. If I can't, then you can sign the paper saying it was necessary, in your opinion."

"Be sure and write down that we tried to find the parents," said Zaorski.

"Trust me."

"I trust everybody. I just wanna cut the deck."

Zaorski put on sterile gloves and cut into Pamela's foot, complaining the whole time about the constantly multiplying rules that hospitals are initiating to protect themselves against lawsuits.

"It's getting ridiculous. We might as well have a lawyer standing beside us. So's malpractice insurance. I understand it costs $9,000 a year premium in Los Angeles. Plastic guys get socked the worst. Patients scream, 'Look what you did to my nose, you bastard,' and sue you for $12 million."

When there was a period of almost an hour without a page or a summons from Shirley, Zaorski relaxed with a couple of other doctors on night duty. They were talking about Cooley, his skill, his money—a continuing topic of conversation among the younger men.

One doctor began doing mental arithmetic and announced that Cooley was potentially the highest-paid doctor in the world. "Look at it this way," he said, scribbling with his ball-point pen on the leg of his scrub suit. "He does 1,000 pump cases a year at $1,500 each, that's $1.5 million. Plus another half million, easy, from his vessel work. That's $2 million if he collects from everybody."

Zaorski disagreed. "But he knocks a lot of fees off. I saw him throw six unpaid bills in the wastebasket at one sitting."

"He's gotta be worth $10 million, easily."

"In medical school," Zaorski said, "we learned that a good surgeon can make up to $75,000 a year in a small town and maybe $100,000 to $300,000 in the city."

"Why is Cooley so good?" I asked, blinded by the tally sheet on the doctor's pants.

"Speed's the main thing," said Zaorski. "It's so important in these cases. If you keep a patient on the pump too long, his blood loses the ability to clot and he can become acidotic—that's an abundance of lactic acid. Just before a patient dies, he fills up with this stuff. Speed is the difference between success and failure in open-heart work. Cooley even got down to where he could do a heart transplant in 36 minutes."

"But they're all dead," said the doctor standing at the coffee pot.

"Yeah," said Zaorski. "That's right. Transplants are a stupid way of doing things."

CHAPTER
7

Seventy-two hours after surgery, Pamela was sitting up, sipping a Coke, brushing her hair, and tearing into get-well cards. The bluish cast to her skin was gone, the sadness had slipped from her eyes, and though she was still pale, there was a general *alive*ness about her that had not been there before Cooley rearranged her heart. Leachman listened to her heart and she accepted his stethoscope without protest. "You must be sick, Pammy, you're so quiet," he said, nodding encouragingly at her mother. "There's still a lot of getting-used-to necessary for the lungs," he said later. "It'll be a few months before those hissing noises go away, but I believe she's going to be fine."

Carstairs went from Recovery to the sixth-floor Intensive Care Unit, where his vital signs were observed for 36 hours, then on to a semiprivate room, where his roommate was disturbing him more than the postoperative pain. The man in the next bed was an 81-year-old farmer, Leroy Castle, who had had a variety of surgery, some vessel work, his gall bladder removed. From a town so small it was not even on the map, he was confused by the hospital and fought off the sedatives given him. When awake he talked constantly in a booming hog-calling voice and was visited frequently by eight large relatives, all of whom talked louder than he did, and all at once. "I thought it was bad in ICU when a man died in the next bed," said Carstairs. "They pulled the curtains around his cubicle, but I knew what was happening. This is worse. I can't get any rest."

Castle was at that moment accusing the nurses of stealing his suitcase. "It's right here, Mr. Castle," said a weary black nurse. "Lemme see it, I don't believe you," roared the farmer. He was trying to stand up in bed on shaky old legs and the nurse was torn between fetching his suitcase from the closet and making him lie down. She chose the latter and threatened to tie his arms to the bed unless he behaved. "I'm gonna call the mayor *and* the sheriff," he said. "I'm gonna tell somebody how the cow ate the cabbage." The nurse sighed and went to the closet and pulled out his beat-up cardboard grip. She held it up above her head so Mr. Castle could see it. "Lemme just touch it," he said. The nurse walked over to his bed. The old man, with surprising strength, snatched it from her and tried to smuggle it under his sheet. The nurse dived after it and put it on his dresser. "I'll leave it here so you can see it," she said. "Now, Mr. Castle, stop misbehaving and get some rest. You want to get out of here, don't you?"

Quiet and still just long enough for the nurse to leave the room, Mr. Castle jumped up and shouted, "All I want to do is leave and go out to a restaurant and get a real dinner! I promise to come back!"

"If it wasn't for that," whispered Carstairs, jerking his thumb toward the next bed, "I'd be fine. Poor old fellow—I guess he's lonely. I asked for a private room and they said they'd move me later today." He touched his hand to his chest, where the incision was held together with sutures and wire brads. "I haven't breathed so well in years. I think I can actually feel the blood circulating in my body." His wife took his hand and kissed it and held it tightly against her face. "I can remember the nights when he would fall asleep and gasp for breath," she said, "and I would lie there with my eyes open until dawn, terrified."

Farmer Castle had probably been slightly senile before his surgery, but his postoperative course had confused him even more. It was an infrequent occurrence but one which, until it cleared up within a few days, was disturbing to all concerned. Elderly patients often get "squirrely," as one anesthesiologist put it, from any drug, even aspirin. Something as powerful as anesthesia can scramble their senses.

A second potential peril is a tiny bubble of air—an embolism—which can swim to the brain and cause convulsion, twitching, disorientation, even death. When the heart is opened for repair, air floods in. When the surgeon closes the heart, he tries to withdraw all the air. Various surgeons have favorite methods of accomplishing this. Cooley draws air out with a syringe, DeBakey tips the end of the operating table down, others blow carbon dioxide gas all over the field. But sometimes a bubble remains and causes trouble.

The Recovery Room and Intensive Care Unit are sometimes severe experiences for patients, particularly the elderly ones. "ICU produces psychoses in some people," said the anesthesiologist. It may well be the loss of the day-night cycle. After surgery, patients wake up in a room that is strange to them, where there are no windows, where the lights are always on, where they do not know the time. It is a world of monitoring machines and beeping noises and crises in the next cubicle.

There is more drama to be found in St. Luke's Recovery than the rest of the hospital, a continuing drama of compression and spontaneity, because at any given moment there are up to 24 patients (half on Cooley's service) crowded three feet from each other. Each patient is in intense pain, each is demanding consolation and attention as he makes the journey from object to being. It takes a special breed of nurse to cope with the extraordinary physical—and emotional—demands of Recovery. The room, originally designed for Central Supply, is low-ceilinged and oppressive and, with patients struggling to climb out of their beds or yank the vital tubes and wires from their bodies, the atmosphere is, at times, that of the battlefield hospital in *M.A.S.H.* The care dispensed is professional and good, but rationed out by a small, overworked, and sometimes testy staff. When a patient pulled out his nose tube and the male nurse wearily stuck it back in again, the patient yelled, "I'm gonna take it out again, it's killing me." "You do that," snapped the nurse, "and I'll put in a bigger one." One disoriented patient spent an entire day fighting everyone until his arms were finally restrained with white furry stays. Seeing a doctor attending the patient in the next bed, the patient used his only available weapon, the right foot, and kicked the doctor in the ribs. The doctor spun around with a fist clenched and fury in his eyes. For one breathless moment the charge nurse thought she was going to see a doctor hit a patient. "I'm sorry," he said, putting his fist down, "It must be the Ben Taub syndrome." He referred to his several months in the Emergency Room of the charity hospital, where young doctors, on occasion, have had to knock down mean drunks or else find themselves with a missing tooth.

The major event of every operating day is at 7 P.M., when the relatives are allowed into Recovery for a few minutes to see the patient after his surgery. There is nothing sicker-looking in medicine than a postoperative major surgery case, with chest painted a ghastly orange, wrapped generously in bandages and tape, covered with wires and tubes through which inch blood and urine. Not infrequently a wife sees a husband and has to be led screaming from the room. About once a week a mother keels over in a faint at first glimpse of her perfectly recovering child. The parents of heart babies have a grueling time. They have not slept at all the night before surgery, have spent ten paralyzing hours in the waiting room, and when at last permitted to see what the surgeon has wrought, cannot cope with the sight.

Ever since the advent of open-heart surgery in 1955, psychiatrists have been running studies on the attendant emotional problems. The incidence of postoperative psychoses in some groups studied has run as high as 25 percent of all patients. Ideally, each candidate for open-heart surgery should be thoroughly examined and evaluated by a psychiatrist to determine if he is emotionally able to withstand the operation and the hours thereafter. But in Houston, there are too many patients, not enough time. Neither Cooley nor DeBakey feels the occasional psychosis is as important as the principal fact of the case: that the heart needs and will get repair.

By Sunday night, Recovery was eerily empty. All the patients of the week had progressed from Recovery upstairs to Intensive Care then to their rooms and, hopefully, to discharge in seven or eight days. Ten years ago, heart patients stayed in the hospital from six weeks to two months; in 1970 the average stay was down to ten days. "Denton really cuts 'em up, sews 'em up, and moves 'em out," said a colleague with a voice sitting on the fence between admiration and derision. The shortened stay could be credited to many things—better pumps, improved anesthesia and its use, the years of experience for all members of the team—but nothing counted as heavily as the dazzling speed and drive of the surgeon-in-chief.

On Monday morning, the deserted Recovery began filling up—fast. Cooley plunged into a schedule of twelve cases, including two double-valve replacements and two coronary artery bypasses, the operation he was not supposed to like to do. He passed by the schedule board on his way to Room 1, and I stopped him with a question. "Do you ever wonder if the sick people will stop coming? That someday you will have repaired all the bad hearts?"

"I certainly hope not," he said. "And so do my creditors."

Dr. Shafi, a dark, good-looking Iranian surgeon had ward duty this morning, meaning he would be tending to patients and not participating in surgery. None of the fellows looked forward to ward duty, no more than any of them relished night call. All wanted to spend as much time as possible scrubbed in, standing next to Cooley. All were disappointed when they came to Houston and discovered that they would not be doing any actual heart surgery, only opening, first-assisting, and closing. "Does it ever get boring?" I asked Shafi. He was in the coffee room waiting for the operator to page him and send him off somewhere to diagnose a spiked fever or take out stitches or write prescriptions for patients anxious to be dismissed.

"Sure," he said. "But not to D.A.C. He is driven by the numbers. A thousand pumps in six months . . . 2,000 in one year. He wants to break his own record. And maybe break"—Shafi threw a thumb in the direction of Methodist—"him."

During the coronary operation that took place shortly after lunch—lunch being a term to indicate time, because Cooley does not stop for it, never more than a sandwich on the fly—he began sewing in the artery taken from the thigh, tediously affixing it to the aorta. He looked up and said to the room, "You practice for this procedure by circumcising gnats."

Late in the long afternoon—it was going to be well into the night before Cooley finished and could make rounds—some of the fellows were quietly discussing something when I walked into the coffee room. There was stiff silence. They did not want me to hear what they were talking about. Suddenly the conversation shifted to Dr. Tanaka, the stocky, muscled Japanese who had to put up with ribbing almost every day of his year in Houston.

"Tanaka," fibbed Shafi, "has a new procedure for opening the chest cavity. He doesn't use a scalpel. He kicks open the patient with karate."

During the laughter, John Zaorski stormed into the coffee lounge. He ripped off his mask and threw it into the garbage can overflowing with coffee cups. He sat down on the couch to dictate an operation summary. "Shit," he said, before he pressed down the dictation button. "You work for three hours trying to get a guy's heart started and nothing happens. Nothing!"

Unknowingly Zaorski had revealed what I was not supposed to hear. Grady Hallman had been doing a coronary in Room 1, and the patient had died on the table. For most of the afternoon, the team—with help from Cooley who had come into the room—struggled to resuscitate him.

"We couldn't get him off the pump," said Zaorski. "Cooley recommended everything in the book, but nothing worked."

"Did you shock him?" someone asked.

"Ten times. Maybe twenty." Zaorski began the dreary recital of a man's last hours. A few days later, a stenographer would send the report to the dead man's home-town doctor. When he finished, Zaorski rubbed his cheeks with his hands for a while. "Thank God it doesn't happen very often—once a month most, maybe every two months. At some hospitals—every day."

The patient was brought on the rolling stretcher to the corridor just inside surgery and a folding green screen was placed around him. People lowered their eyes as they passed by. Cooley went to his office, dictated a letter, and returned to surgery, stopping at the box full of masks for a new one. The death was on his mind. "This time, I wasn't going to go searching for a donor heart," he said in a voice curiously flat and one-note. "I decided to let him die in peace."

Half an hour later the fellows were joking, not for the fun therein, but in an attempt to erase the defeat. One of the young surgeons suggested: "Write on the chart that Zaorski was first-assisting and was heavy-handed."

"Heavy-handed!" Zaorski yelled. "You couldn't change a tire and you call me heavy-handed!"

The body was taken downstairs for a post-mortem and picked up by a funeral home, which would handle the lucrative local embalming and arrange for transportation to the man's home town. "They come right away," said Zaorski. "They're anxious to get their hands on the corpse."

Time began to blur the faces and fates of the patients, the days and nights welding together. I would store patients in my mind, promising to get back to them, but new ones kept crowding them out and the old ones vanished. By the time I remembered that interesting atrial septal defect—names were lost as well, only the diseases stuck—that interesting ASD was gone, dismissed, well, or dead, on his way home, or already there.

Carstairs checked out before I could say good-bye; Pamela was leaving on a morning when I was on the children's heart floor to see somebody else.

"How do you feel, Pammy?"

"Fine," she said shyly, flipping up her nightgown automatically to show her scar, healing well. It would fade into a thin white line within a few months.

Mrs. Kroger said she was going to have a genetic study done on her family. "And tell my daughters the history of our heart disease. I hope they don't ever have to go through the hell of this."

The skill and achievement of the heart surgeon is most dramatically seen in the juxtaposition of two facts:

1. Before 1955, when the heart-lung machine was developed, most babies born with serious cardiovascular defects either died at birth or lived a drastically shortened, terror-filled life.

2. By 1970, only fifteen years later, the heart surgeon could repair and promise normal life to upwards of 80 percent of congenitally

damaged hearts. It is an achievement in medicine that ranks with Pasteur, Fleming, and Salk. But there are still the other 20 percent:

Grady Hallman began a tricky case on a ten-month-old baby girl named Kimberly born with a ventricular septal defect, complicated with subaortic stenosis—a thickening of the lower aorta. This is one of the few congenital defects that must be operated on definitively; there is no palliative operation to tide a baby over until it is older and stronger. "She wouldn't live to her first birthday without this operation," said John Zaorski.

The procedure would not begin for a quarter hour or so; Zaorski and I went to the lounge to have coffee. There were half a dozen conversations going on at once. I stood in the doorway tuning in and out as a man flips a radio dial.

"God help me to never go through that again," the resident fresh from DeBakey's service was saying. "He would stand there at the table and rap me on the knuckles with the needle holder and tell the room, 'Wants to be a cardiovascular surgeon, wants to be a cardiovascular surgeon, but he performs like a brick layer.' I didn't have the courage to tell him I *never* wanted to be a cardiovascular surgeon."

Two doctors were talking of an article in *Life* magazine that told of a Midwestern town with a new hospital and no doctor to run it, despite the guarantee that such a man could earn at least $40,000 a year. "You can earn $75,000 a year," said John Russell dryly, "giving flu shots, insurance examinations, and writing excuses for people to stay home from work."

"You take these guys out of surgery," a pediatric surgeon was saying to a girl student, referring to Cooley and DeBakey, "and put them in business or industry, and they'd be Ross Perot or Bernie Cornfeld. Wait, make that Tom Watson or Henry Ford."

"Industry?" said the student.

"You think it's *not* an industry? I mean, the by-products are great —people get cured, people get caught, but it's still an industry."

"That's a helluva case, that baby," said Zaorski. He had been transferred to another room at the last minute but had watched Hallman begin the ventricular septal defect and subaortic stenosis. "I don't think the kid's gonna make it."

In Room 1, Hallman was trying to get the baby's heart to respond. Lola, the scrub nurse, had normally mischievous eyes, but now they were wide and saddened. Hallman fought to activate the heart for more than an hour. He shocked it over and over again. He unclamped the tubes and took the infant off the pump and the heart refused to beat. He put her back on the pump and things seemed to work. But when he shocked her and took her off the pump, the heart refused to beat. Cooley came over from Room 2, where he was doing a valve and said, "Has Nora been told? Better find him, it's his case." Nora was Dr. James Nora, a staff pediatric cardiologist.

"I've already told the parents it's not going very well," said Cooley, backing out of the room and returning to his valve.

Another nurse pushed open the doors in the middle of the struggle and said, "Dr. Hallman, the amputation patient in Room 3 is ready."

"Go ahead and put him to sleep." Hallman's hands were inside the heart of the dying baby.

"He *is* asleep."

"Then drape him."

"He *is* draped."

"Then find Dr. Messmer [Dr. Bruno Messmer, a Swiss surgical fellow] and see if he can start it."

Three hours into an operation that should have taken half that, Hallman lifted his hands with a great slowness from the heart and shook his head. Nothing was said. No pronouncement was made. He only shook his head. There was no point in going further. Nora had come in and seen the futility of it all and went out to find the parents. Hallman left the room; somebody would sew her up. One of the pump technicians bumped into the heart-lung machine and a container of blood flowed sadly across the green tile.

A chaplain was sent to find the child's parents. They were led, fearful, to the family room not far from surgery where Nora told them. Sometimes parents rail and scream and attack the surgeon when a child is lost. Parents have lunged at Cooley and beat his breast until their hands are sore, but he never moves. The couple who had brought the child to the hospital, were both twenty-one, both incredibly young. They took the news with dignity. Only Nora's eyes were clouded and he was rubbing them when he left the room.

Bill Murrah, the student chaplain from Alabama on a summer internship at St. Luke's from Union Seminary in New York, leaned against the wall outside. "There's not much you can tell them," he said. "They don't want any religious formulas or quotations from the Bible at a time like this. They just want to know if their baby is alive or dead, and if she is dead, would she have lived *without* the surgery. They all want to know that, they need desperately to be told 'NO' so they won't feel like accomplices."

Lola, the scrub nurse, hurried into the nurse's locker room to dress and go pick up her four-year-old son who was staying at a nursery near the Medical Center. "All I want to do is hide in the bathroom," she said. "Nobody'll ever know I had anything to do with that precious baby's death. The first patient I ever scrubbed on died . . . a Fallot. . . . That's when I quit. For the first time." A child's death sends a shock wave through the women of the heart team.

One of the motherly-type nurses picked up Kim from the operating table and wrapped her in a pink and yellow blanket and took her out to the surgical corridor, where a rolling baby crib was standing, the same bed in which she had been brought—with her mother leaning over her—to the operating room, the same bed in which two pink diaper pins and a pacifier were waiting for her. The nurse pulled a green sheet across her baby and in a few moments, a coordinating nurse from Texas Children's gently took her and carried her by hand to the morgue.

Another child was on a rolling bed in the surgical corridor as the coordinating nurse walked by. She had a curious pinched face and she refused to laugh at Dr. Girgis, the Egyptian-born anesthesiologist who was taking used surgical gloves and blowing them up like balloons and drawing faces on them with his felt pen. He had almost filled up her bed with the cheerful faces but she was not a child who knew how to laugh.

"We'll save these for you," he said. "You can play with them tomorrow."

The child told me her name was Joy and that she was the daughter of a truck driver from Oregon. She was eight, she said, but she looked half that. The blueness of her Tetralogy of Fallot made her appear cold.

There was a depression buried within me, and it had been roused
with the baby's death. I was weary of the hospital and its surgery. My
own son, my second son, would be coming from his home in New
York to spend the summer with me. Despite his strong body, despite
his ability to plant his skis together and take the *plus difficiles* runs in
the French Alps or plow into his older brother in Central Park carrying a football, his heart had something wrong with it. Nine years ago
he had been born in this very Houston hospital and the pediatrician
had heard a murmur—not a grave murmur—but a worrying, hissing
echo that vibrated the tiny chambers. Cardiologists in New York
and France had listened to it in the years that followed. They kept
saying that he should be examined every year or two, but that his
life need not be restricted. "Do not tell him about the murmur," the
doctor in New York had said. "Don't let him favor it." I had planned
to have him examined by Cooley's staff, but—had an operation been
indicated that afternoon, if there was talk of the knife—I could not
have signed the paper to deliver him into a surgeon's hands. I dressed
and left the hospital. I found a movie to erase two hours. I telephoned
New York and spoke with my son Scott, who was full of plans for his
return to Texas. I hung up and called the hospital; its lure was not to
be denied. John Zaorski had night duty again and he was brusque.
Things were, he said, frantic.

I found him in Recovery. "I've gotta go tell a man his wife just
died," he said. He was writing a death certificate. In the corner,
nurses were pulling drapes around the bed of an elderly woman who
had had a double valve replacement the day before. She had arrived
at St. Luke's in grave heart failure, bubbling from the fluids in her
lungs and chest. "She was almost dead before the operation," Zaorski said. "I went down and told her husband about an hour ago that
she wasn't doing well, so he's prepared." Death messages were normally given in two stages. If the patient died during surgery, Cooley
or a fellow went out and said that the operation was not going well,
that serious problems had arisen, that there was little hope—even
though the patient was already lost and being sewn up. Then, half an
hour, an hour later, the final news was delivered. "It's easier that
way," said Zaorski. "On us and on them."

The neatly dressed old man was in the Family Room. He looked up, unable to control the twitches in his unshaven cheeks. "I'm sorry," said Zaorski immediately upon entering the room. "We did everything we could. But she's gone. . . ."

Instantly the old man wept, silently, ashamedly. He apologized for his tears. Zaorski intruded tactfully on his grief. "There's just one more thing," he said. "We'd like to examine her heart. We can maybe learn better why she died."

"I don't object to that," said the new widower. "If her death could help anybody else. . . ."

On the long walk back to the coffee room, I asked about Joy, the child who had followed the baby into surgery.

"Who?" asked Zaorski, searching his mental list of the day's surgery.

"Joy, the last little girl, the Fallot."

"Oh. She died on the table."

"Two in one day on the same table?"

"Yeah. Couldn't get her off the pump." Zaorski walked on with his head down. Was his shield cracking, or was he too much of a tyro at the business to have one? "Sometimes," he said, "this is a lousy service . . . sometimes it's worse than a leukemia ward."

He telephoned Pathology and reported permission for the woman's post. "It's been a rough night," he said later in the coffee room. "Just before you came, there was a STAT call on sixth-floor ICU." (STAT is short for the Latin "statum," which means "immediately" but in hospital code it means "emergency.") An 86-year-old woman with a pacemaker had arrested and when Zaorski got there the nurse had her on the respirator and somebody else was massaging her chest. Zaorski hooked up the cardiac press and put an endotracheal tube down her throat, the kind with a balloon attached to the end of it. Once the tube gets down, the doctor pumps on the balloon and it stops air from going to the stomach and pushes it directly into the lungs. Zaorski also shot adrenalin into the heart. But the scope stayed flat. Nothing would bring her back.

"This may be the Tet offensive tonight," said Zaorski. "They'll be dropping from the trees."

Shirley, the Recovery nurse, rushed in near midnight with her half-smile that concealed worry. She had the chart of a young Italian woman named Vincenza who had appeared at St. Luke's looking like a concentration-camp survivor. Vincenza had sunken cheeks to which she applied bright, heavy rouge, giving her face the appearance of a death mask. She weighed but 78 pounds and she had Ebstein's Disease, a rare defect of the tricuspid valve that few surgeons would touch. Cooley had put in a new valve and now Shirley suspected tamponade, bleeding around the heart. There was no urine output to speak of either.

"All right," said Zaorski. When Shirley was worried, John followed through. As Zaorski was leaving, a young brunette ward nurse interrupted him. She had an expression of absolute exasperation on her face.

"It's Mr. Castle," she said. The old farmer had been transferred from the semiprivate room, where he had been keeping Carstairs awake, to the ward for disturbed elderly patients down the hall.

"What's Mr. Castle doing?"

"He's disoriented, climbing out of bed, yelling, disturbing half the floor."

"Tell me something new. What did you give him?"

"Thorazine and Demerol," said the nurse. "But he's still very much with us."

"How much Demerol?"

"Thirty-five milligrams."

"Give him 50 more."

The nurse looked startled. "I don't want to pile all that Demerol into an 81-year-old man."

"Look," said Zaorski, impatiently. "What's Demerol going to do at worst—depress the blood pressure, right? You've gotta depress him, or he's gonna kill himself."

"Okay." The nurse gave in.

"Did you tie him down?"

"Hours ago."

"I'll be by to see him."

Zaorski went into Recovery first, where the emaciated Italian girl, perspiring heavily, was almost lost in the bed. He looked at her x-rays. Shirley slapped them onto the viewer and winced in pain. The nurse had bursitis, aggravated from reaching up so often to put the x-rays in place. Zaorski ordered digitalis and a plasma-type fluid for Vincenza.

"If I give her more blood," he told Shirley, "it'll thicken up the blood she already has, and make it even tougher to get it circulating. Which is what she needs." He did not buy Shirley's suspicion of tamponade.

In the disturbed patients ward, Mr. Castle had kicked over his intravenous stand several times and was generally driving the ward nurse up the wall. His favorite trick was to wiggle down to the middle of the bed, drape his legs over the end, and kick, as vigorously as a child learning to swim. The nurse would lug him back to where his head touched the pillow and scold him, and as soon as she turned her back, he would wiggle back again. She had finally tied his hands firmly to the rails with white furry straps that could not cut him.

"Poor old guy, he's screwed up. This sometimes happens when the cardiac output fails." Zaorski watched him struggle against the retaining straps. "He'll be all right."

Within half an hour, Vincenza's urine tube was beginning to fill, a sure sign that the digitalis and plasma were working and that the heart was pumping strongly enough to support the kidneys. "Score one for our side," said Zaorski. He noticed that Shirley was still in pain from the bursitis; he persuaded her to take a cortisone shot and permit him to bind her arm to her waist. "Trust Dr. Zaorski," he said. "Keep it that way and the pain'll go away in a day or so."

Hospitals normally quiet down after midnight but not this night. A fat woman cried out all night with gall bladder pain; Zaorski went to see her twice and agreed that she probably hurt, but not enough to wake up the whole floor. Another Italian, a woman in her mid-twenties named Maria Celestina, was causing her usual trouble. Hers was one of the more interesting cases on Cooley's service. A pretty, vivacious girl, she had fallen down a well in her village when she was a child and developed a traumatic aneurysm of the thoracic area. Surgeons in Italy had wrapped it with cellophane, but it had grown worse over the years and she had come to Houston. Cooley had excised the aneurysm and replaced it with a Dacron graft. She seemed to be recovering satisfactorily in her room, but she was still a bit goofy and considerably lonely. The only English phrase she felt comfortable with was "Please help me" and she sang it and moaned it with orchestration. What she mainly wanted was company. The fel-

lows had all learned her trick; she would exhort, "Please help me" as
one passed by her open door. If he succumbed to the lure and went to
see if anything was the matter, she would beckon for him to come
close to the bed and try to grab him.

Maria Celestina started warbling "Please help me" in Puccini fashion close to 3 A.M. but Zaorski was too tired to do anything but slam
her door shut, firmly, as he went to see about quieting down Mr.
Castle for the fourth time.

The week was disastrous. "We go through long periods when nothing happens," said one of the fellows in the coffee room the next
morning. "Weeks when everybody gets well, months when nobody
dies, nobody even bleeds around a graft, then we get a week like this
and I'd like to switch to dermatology."

Cooley was doing a routine valve replacement later that day when
one of the stunning mysteries of cardiac work occurred. At St.
Luke's it is called "stone heart" for lack of a better name. The patient's
left ventricle suddenly went into a spasm, not unlike a Charley Horse
in the leg, and nothing yet known to medicine could bring it back or
save the patient. Neither the origin nor the cause is known.

"It's almost like witchcraft," said Jerry Strong. "It could be something muscular, or pollution in the air, or a fall in the stock market
for all we know." Cooley said he has not seen more than a dozen
cases in the past decade, and autopsy reveals nothing because the
spasm is over by then. "I used to think it might be due to some pump
defect, but I've dismissed that idea," he said.

As he always does when the rarity occurs, Strong injected all manner of medication into the patient's intravenous, hoping that something
or some combination of something would stop the spasm and allow
the heart to function. But nothing worked. "When it happens,"
Strong said, "they're dead. Period. I must have dumped twenty different kinds into him. I personally think we ought to put all known
medicines into one jug, label it Lazarene, stick it in him, and pray."

About 6:30 that night John Zaorski had ducked down to the basement cafeteria and was well into a Salisbury steak when over the
chatter of the room he heard a faint page. "Cooley Fellow, Three

North, STAT. Cooley Fellow, Three North, STAT." Some hospitals page
Dr. Blue, but the meaning is universal: a heart has arrested and there
are but a handful of moments before it becomes permanent death.

In mid-bite Zaorski dropped his fork, bolted out of the cafeteria,
almost bumping into two nurses weaving their way through the
crowd. For a big man he could move fast, side-stepping the "CAU-
TION—Wet Floor" signs, which made the central corridor an obstacle
course.

The patient was a frail, blue old woman who was stretched out on
a reclining lounge chair beside her bed. Her mouth was gaping,
her eyes were dilated. She was dead. Zaorski picked her up and flung
her like a rag doll onto the bed and began the rhythmic pushing on her
chest. (The tabloid-familiar custom of slicing into chests and massaging hearts is passé; superior results can be obtained with closed-
chest massage.) A young inhalation therapist tore into the room at
the same moment and clamped a breathing bag over her mouth. The
nurse stood there chattering away, stunned by the whole affair. "She
was fine, she was *just* fine. She had her dinner, she saw the doctor,
she was sitting in the chair looking out the window and watching the
TV"—the set was still on, droning out a comedy—"I looked in and
saw she was gone and I pushed the chair back so she'd lie flat and I
sent out a STAT call."

Zaorski nodded but was paying little attention. The look on his
face revealed frustration; his pushing and the therapist's squeezing
seemed to be having no effect at all, and time was running out. Suddenly, almost magically, the old woman's chest heaved, she gasped,
she choked, and back she came from death. "She's on her own!"
Zaorski cried triumphantly. "Let's get her into Recovery." The
nurse turned to find a stretcher, but he stopped her. "Let's just keep
her on the bed," he said, abruptly pushing the end out into the hall.
With the therapist on the other end, the procession sped through the
surgical waiting room—where the families, startled, were lined up
to go in at seven and see the patients—and into Recovery, where a
swarm of doctors hooked her up to the machines and monitors.

Several days later, the woman, a tough, chipper Bostonian, was
preparing to leave the hospital and return home. She had no memory
of the incident other than waking up in Recovery, a place where she
had been ten days previous, after her heart surgery, and a place she

had grown to dislike. "I must have fainted," she said, and the nurse nodded. No one ever remembered those moments on the other side. One woman suffered more than 30 cardiac arrests during her three days in Intensive Care Unit. Flat EKGs, the works. Each time the doctors and nurses would bang on her chest and resuscitate her and each time she would rouse and murmur, "Did I have another one of my sinking spells?" Once she came to just in time to see the nurse preparing to hit her chest and she said, with insult, "And I thought you were my friend."

Happily, Maria Celestina quieted down for a while after a quarter of an hour trans-Atlantic telephone conversation with her sister in Italy—a poignant, sobbing, laughing, sometimes hysterical conversation. Everybody on Three North shared her pleasure.

But sadly, Mr. Castle threw a clot to his brain and died that night in the senile ward. It upset the nurse who had been contending with him. "I wish they had left the old man alone," she said, moping around the nursing station. She was a young registered nurse who had not experienced the loss of many patients. "He was such a nice old man, he was eighty-one, and he'd never been in a hospital before and I had to help him make a phone call to his family because he'd never even had a telephone in his house. He was telling them to be sure and water his tomato plants."

Cooley stayed in his operating rooms from sunrise to sunset, almost as if one death could be assuaged by fixing two more hearts. He betrayed no emotion, no public tears, most likely no private ones. A friend said he was "*un*-emotional." He was, surely, affected by the complications and the run of deaths. "There is no more heat anywhere in medicine than in heart surgery," observed Don Bricker, who had been through the DeBakey program, had operated across from Cooley, and who was now heading surgery at Ben Taub. "There's simply no area of surgery where you can lose patients on the table as you do in heart work. Gun shots, traffic-crushed victims —these patients may crater on you. But with elective heart surgery, *you're* the guy who makes the decision to operate, and when *you* fix the heart and it doesn't start up again, then *you're* the guy who killed him. When it happens to me, I go out and sit somewhere and weep."

Months later, on a Saturday morning in his office, Cooley and I would talk about death. I had never seen a crack in his shield, not even a shadow across his face. How did he hide, or was there anything to hide? "I think I've built a shield," he answered. "One of the big problems, it seems to me, is how the surgeon deals with his disappointments. How to deal with his personal errors, shortcomings, poor judgment, or the complete and total failure which is death. I've observed other surgeons who just take it in their stride, the 'well-we've-done-our-best-school.' I have not been capable of taking it that way. Perhaps you just don't see it within me. But what can I do? You've got to go on, that is the only way to overcome disappointment. Continue your work and realize you are doing good. The tragedy comes when you get two or three bad ones at once and you stop and you start to wondering if you're doing the world any good at all. . . ."

"Do you ever wonder that?"

He shook his head firmly and negatively.

At the end of the bad week, someone remarked that it had been reminiscent of the transplant era, of the saddening days when the first batch of Cooley's transplants, six apparently healthy and rejuvenated people, all started rejecting and dying, and rather than stop, rather than a moratorium, Cooley did more and more. Eight became twelve, fifteen turned into twenty. "His hands had never failed him," said a friend. "And he couldn't understand it."

But any confidence misplaced or temporarily lost during the transplant year had long since come back. Cooley seems to feel that if *he* cannot help a patient in the operating room, if *his* hands cannot find and hold the spark of life, then it simply cannot be done. "Denton knows when he has done a good operation," observed a senior member of his team. "But he doesn't go to all extremes to keep them alive in Recovery or ICU. If they don't get better due to their new hemodynamic situation, then . . ."—the doctor made a hopeless gesture with his upturned hands. "Mike DeBakey, conversely, will go to hell and back to keep the patient alive. If he dies a month later at home—well, the operation was a success. . . ."

At the Saturday morning pathology conference, Cooley talked briefly and dispassionately of the ten-month-old baby Kimberly's death. One case a week is selected for extensive discussion. "It was a most confusing heart," he said. "She had such complete heart block afterward that even a pacemaker wouldn't drive it, and we ended up with a fiasco on our hands." Dr. Rosenberg, the pathologist, took the infant's heart out of a plastic container and put it on a sheet of wrapping paper to give his theories. "The septum was closed, there was a grotesque left ventricle. And note this unusually deep cleft in the mitral valve, which is rapidly becoming our most frequent rarity."

C H A P T E R

8

Something struck me again and again, and though I witnessed it, and heard and thought about it a hundred times, I never understood why —why the passive acceptance, why the offering up of the human heart to this man with fewer words than one would deliver to a splendid mechanic on the subject of a malfunctioning limousine? Twenty times a week, when Cooley entered their rooms on the eve of their surgery, they turned down their television sets and scrooched up on their pillows and the conversations—*invariably*—went like this:

Cooley: (Ambling near) "Well, we think we ought to fix you up tomorrow."

Patient: "Okay."

Cooley: "I'll be out to see your wife [or husband] after the operation."

Patient: "That's what I came here for."

Cooley: "You'll be fine." (Smiling, exiting.)

I have never had a tooth filled without worrying the dentist with questions from the cost of his drill to the identity of the artist who composed the water color above his mixing pots. On the two occasions I underwent minor surgery—a hernia and an appendectomy— I put everyone, scrub maids not excepted, through my inquisition. How can it be otherwise? Is the eve of heart surgery so staggering that one falls mute? Or is it that one becomes timid in the presence of celebrity, as a child would do if suddenly face to face with a baseball player?

I asked Cooley why everyone acquiesced so readily. Fear? Ignorance? Shock? "Blind faith, mainly," he replied. "They've read that it's good and they want to keep that feeling." He was walking down a corridor at the moment with John Russell and they were talking of a child who had been admitted to the hospital for probable surgery, but about whom a decision had not been reached by the pediatric cardiologists. "Most pediatricians I've known are thoughtful and deliberate," Cooley said, "and to the surgeon that means slow."

Leachman catheterized a patient that afternoon who would have seemed to have been the last man alive in need of heart surgery. The very antithesis of Arthur Bingham, he followed all the rules. At 44, Vic Coleman had a strong, finely proportioned physique, still hardened by the football he had played in the Marine Corps V12 program during World War II, later at the University of Southern California, where he starred in the Rose Bowl and got whipped by Alabama—he remembers every play—still later with a professional team at Buffalo in the old All-American Conference, finally with the Rams. He had been a sculptured 215 pounds then, 40 more than his present weight, and he had never suffered a major injury. Since 1951 he had been an oilman in Midland, Texas.

Questioned by Leachman, Coleman said his job was a low-pressure one, that he went to work at eight or nine or whenever he felt like it, and he rarely stayed past four. He did little traveling other than going to the site of a well and sitting around waiting for it to come in. Moreover, he did not smoke, drink, eat butter, eggs, milk, or high cholesterol foods. He took superb care of himself, watched his weight, had a complete medical checkup including an EKG each year, and had never stopped participating in sports. He played tennis in the summer, skied in the winter, even rounded up a group of twenty businessmen and persuaded them to skip the cocktail hour in favor of jogging every afternoon at five. "We did twenty laps—five miles—on the high school track and I was to the point where I could do it in 38 minutes—about seven minutes for one mile." Coleman's father had died of a heart attack at the age of 63, which was the only blemish on an otherwise extraordinary prognosis for the good long life.

"Jesus H. Christ," said one of the fellows after checking him over. "If *he* has heart trouble, we should all be dead from infarcts about six years ago."

But by no means did all the heart doctors subscribe to the recognized guidelines to forestall heart trouble. DeBakey, for one, feels stress is not only acceptable, but "quite good for you." A Houston cardiologist named Dr. Charles Armbrust had one patient who suffered a heart attack and died in the middle of his morning pushups. "And every morning when I'm driving to the hospital," said Dr. Armbrust, "I see an elderly man and his elderly dog jogging beside the road. I keep wondering who is going to infarct first—the dog or his master."

The matter of cholesterol had long divided those involved in heart work. No doctor would deny the value of a low cholesterol diet—for one thing, it lowers calories and would tend to keep the patient slim and reduce the amount of work the heart must do. But no one has ever proved that reducing cholesterol intake in an adult's diet has anything to do with reducing the danger of a heart attack!

Coleman's trouble had come suddenly, less than three months earlier, when he had been jogging and felt sharp chest pains just under his rib cage. "The pain kept boiling up for days after," he told Leachman, "but I passed it off. Then I went skiing and fell on my pole, which made the pain worse. I thought I'd cracked a rib. I went back to Midland and played three sets of tennis and I could hardly get through them. In the days after that, for the first time in my life, any exertion at all would bring on pain. I couldn't walk a block and a half without it coming on."

"How would you describe the pain?" asked Leachman.

"Like somebody was standing on my chest and wouldn't get off. And I knew my heart was skipping a beat because I checked it regularly with a stethoscope. I always had. It was crazy, it ran like an old John Deere tractor. It'd go one-two-three-skip, or sometimes it would go up to fourteen and then skip three times."

A hometown doctor diagnosed angina pectoris and informed Coleman that he could live for years by popping nitro tablets—but that it would mean a drastic if not total curtailing of his passion for sport. "I'd just as soon be dead," he said. "I charged down to the University of Texas Medical Center in Galveston, where this specialist wanted to do a Vineburg* on me. Then I heard that Cooley was doing this bypass operation up in Houston and five minutes after I heard about it, I knew I had to get up here and have it done. It's a shame I had to get heart trouble, but if I've got it, let's get the game on and get it over with."

The cardiograms showed that Coleman was the classic candidate for the bypass: a man in his mid-forties with obstruction high up in the right coronary artery. He had not progressed to the point of advanced arterial disease which would have made it difficult for the surgeon to sew in the leg vein. And, ideally, he had extreme pain, the one thing that can usually be improved by the procedure.

I asked cardiologist Don Rochelle why Coleman had been stricken. With not a visible misdemeanor on his medical records, what hope was there for those of us who commit compound felonies?

"I guess he just has an inability to handle fat within his body," said Rochelle. "We all try to avoid cholesterol, but what the lay public doesn't realize is that two-thirds to three-fourths of it is manufactured within the body and not brought in by diet. The pure form of this is definitely inherited."

Cooley scheduled Coleman for a coronary bypass the next day, and when informed of his patient's extraordinary health regime, said dryly, "The trouble is, his grandfather wasn't castrated."

---

* *The Vineburg is a coronary operation pioneered by a Canadian doctor and now totally out of favor at the Houston hospitals. It consisted of tunneling the mammary artery to the heart and hoping for a new blood supply. The trouble was that it took three months to become functional—time enough for someone with heart disease to have another heart attack—and the flow of blood was less than 10 cc's per minute, about one-tenth that of normal coronary arterial flow.*

Late that afternoon one of the residents from DeBakey's program trudged into the St. Luke's coffee room looking one-third sheepish, one-third frightened, and one-third hysterical. He sat down and, explaining his presence in the alien camp, said, "I just got thrown out of DeBakey's operating room."

"What'd you do?" asked John Zaorski.

"He said I made the sutures too long." The resident's name was Geoff and he was a red-haired father of four. Zaorski shook his head in sympathy and disbelief. A third-year medical student learns how to put in sutures; by the time a doctor reaches his third year of surgical residency—with eleven years of medical training behind him—there could be little question as to his ability in sewing up wounds. Geoff was considered one of the more promising heart surgeons in Houston; the very real peril he faced was that with little more than one month remaining on the academic year, he would not get credit for the year unless he somehow found his way back into DeBakey's good will. A senior member of DeBakey's staff had advised Geoff to stay low for a few days and then drift back in. "Usually he'll miss you in the middle of an operation and growl for you to get scrubbed —quick," said the older man, who had seen the trauma before and knew what to prescribe.

Leachman heard of Geoff's trouble and grimaced. "Well, he isn't the first resident, nor will he be the last, to get chucked out by Mike. And Mike's too powerful to argue with. He may well be the most powerful physician in America, and that does not exclude the Surgeon-General or the Secretary of Health, Education and Welfare."

Surgery in both hospitals was especially well attended the next several days because the World Cancer Congress was meeting in downtown Houston and scores of surgical delegates slipped away to the Texas Medical Center to watch Cooley and DeBakey. The protocol of such visits has long since been established. It is not unlike travel in the Middle East, in that the traveler can go without trouble from Cairo to Tel Aviv. The Israelis do not care. But it is impossible to go the other way without having two passports. The touring doctor does well to call on Methodist and DeBakey first, and then go the hundred yards to St. Luke's and Cooley, who, in truth, does not mind being the second stop, because he knows that his surgery is dazzling enough for anybody.

Cooley was at the peak of his form for Coleman's coronary artery bypass. Twenty-five doctors jammed the room, including a doctor from India with a floppy nurse's hat covering his pink turban. "This may be the record," said a nurse with some annoyance as she kept pushing visitors out of her view so she could see when Cooley needed, say, the defibrillator paddles. When the anastamosis was finished and Cooley ordered the patient off the pump and Coleman's heart leaped up and began to beat like the finest, truest watch, Zaorski shrewdly asked the head pump technician how long he had been on bypass. She checked the digital timer on the pump and said, "28 minutes." The visitors made looks of approving envy or frank astonishment.

Some surgeons outside Houston who attempt the operation take up to eight hours to accomplish it. Coleman's was only one of eight procedures that Cooley had routinely scheduled for the day, including another coronary bypass immediately afterward. (Christiaan Barnard and other well-known cardiovascular surgeons do only one open-heart case a day, so intense is the emotional and physical strain.)

Zaorski knew that Cooley is proudest of his speed and relished hearing the pump time—the most crucial moments of heart surgery —publicly announced. Had Zaorski, or one of the other fellows failed to pick up the cue, then Cooley himself would probably have asked, and, upon receiving the figure from the head pump technician, would most likely have said, "That long, huh?"

I do not know the boundaries between pride and hubris. But Cooley was later complimented by a delegation of important doctors, including the Surgeon-General of Pakistan, who said, with fervor, "I have never seen surgery like this—anywhere." Cooley, knowing that the man was on a tour of American medical centers, asked, "Where have you been so far?" The Pakistani mentioned several leading hospitals including neighboring Methodist, the Mayo Clinic, and Cornell. "Well," said Cooley, as if that explained everything, "you've been in the backyard."

Once he was showing me around the unfinished surgical floor of the Texas Heart Institute—there would be eight operating rooms, as many as DeBakey had—and he began telling of how difficult it was to raise enormous sums of money and some of the strings people attached. One foundation wanted to name the hospital after Denton Cooley. "I declined," he said. "It won't happen in my lifetime. But a fellow can't control what might come about when he is gone."

Cooley's college friend, the one who still felt uncomfortable in his presence, remarked: "He is a very chauvinistic Texan in which two things merged: Texas pride and his own reputation. These created the edifice we will work in. He sought something permanent by which to be remembered—a bridge, a statue, a hospital."

When Coleman's operation was done, Cooley, trailed by the delegation, went across the hall to perform a coronary bypass on a laundry route foreman from Chicago, who had suffered heart failure a decade previously and a massive coronary two years ago—the reverse of how things usually happen. Doctors in Chicago had told him his heart was so bad that they considered it a 70 percent risk of death to attempt the operation, an 80 percent risk of death if nothing was done at all. "I was between a rock and a hard place," said the foreman. Cooley knocked two minutes off his pump time on this operation, a piece of surgery so exquisite that one of the cancer doctors stood in the room long after Cooley had left and shook his head in amazement.

One of the visitors to the Cancer Congress was obviously well known and respected at St. Luke's because he called Cooley "Denton" and he called Hallman "Grady" and both men made sure he got a favored position at their table. I had glanced at his name tag but it meant nothing to me until John Zaorski tipped me off. He was Dr. James Hardy of the University of Mississippi, a man who three years prior to Christiaan Barnard had performed a surgical feat of stunning magnitude, but which was all but overlooked by the laity. His peers, however, applauded him for it, and he was recognized as one of the world leaders in heart surgery. Hardy was a youngish-looking middle-aged man with a soft Southern accent and that highly charged field of vitality that seems to envelop the surgeon. He was scheduled to deliver a major paper at the Congress the next day but we made a rendezvous for breakfast at 6:30 A.M.

Hardy renewed his amazement at what regularly occurred in Houston. He understood how Cooley could operate on such a schedule because he had no teaching or administrative responsibilities with Baylor. But DeBakey's pace and the breadth of his private practice Hardy could not accept. "I'm chairman of a department of surgery and there are simply not enough hours in a day to do what is expected of me. A chairman's time becomes dissipated. When you become fairly well known, there is a certain amount of national tithing that one must do. And we use the Hopkins system, which is simply that a medical school is there to educate people, not to glorify a surgeon's private practice. There is no way that Mike could function in his manner at our institution. But I suppose we all knew he would become somebody when he dropped in on Dr. Ravdin in Philadelphia about 25 years ago. Ravdin was then the ranking figure of American surgery and one would have expected him to give Mike about ten minutes if he saw him at all. But Mike walked in and spent the whole day. You've got to hand it to Mike and Denton," he said. "Denton is the technician and Mike knew how to spread the news. They've made Houston the heart capital of the world."

From 1956, shortly after the heart-lung bypass pump became available, until 1963, Hardy and his staff did several hundred organ transplants in dogs, swapping kidneys, hearts, and lungs, pointing to the day when a human heart transplant would be possible.

"I realized it would be fraught with enormous emotional overtones. So many people felt the soul dwelt within the heart. I used to ask lay audiences, if they were dying, how many would agree to a kidney transplant to save their life, and a large number would raise their hands. I then asked how many would accept a liver transplant, and a smaller number went up. When I moved to the heart, nobody raised their hand. Nobody.

"The mere fact that we were considering it—working toward it —drew enormous criticism from members of our own institution. The internists thought it was not only immoral but amoral, another surgical prank. If we had waited until the internists were absolutely ready, we wouldn't have gone ahead with kidneys, and thousands of people are alive today due to kidney transplants.

"In late '63 or early '64, we began actively looking for a human recipient in which to implant the heart of a chimpanzee. We were offered numerous potential recipients but they all seemed to be wrong. At that time a human donor had to be, in effect, dead, and the recipient as well. It would have had to have been an extraordinary circumstance, almost an uncanny coincidence, for us to find both donor and recipient at the same moment.

"We felt a chimp's heart was about right physiologically and was as close as we could get to the human organ. Incidentally we paid only $600 for two chimps at that time, and as soon as word got out, doctors all over the country started buying them and overnight the price went up to $1,000 each, and they're $1,500 now, *if* you can find one.

"On January 23, 1964—how well I remember the day—a man named Boyd Rush from Laurel, Mississippi, a man who had had heart trouble for years, was brought into our hospital in shock. We examined him and told his family that there was nothing that could be done for him surgically—but that there was the possibility of a cardiac transplant. We explained that there was a neurological case in the hospital, with the patient near death, and that if death did occur, then we could perhaps use the heart. (I've often since thought that if the situation arose today, the neurosurgeon would simply pull the plug.) But if death did not occur, then would they agree to the heart of a suitable primate? They were less enthusiastic about a 'suitable primate,' but they finally agreed. We told them that if we could improve Mr. Rush's condition to the point where we could explain everything to him, then we would ask him for his consent. But he never reached that state.

"Actually we knew that the chimp heart was vigorous and sound with cardiac output much stronger than either patient Rush or his potential donor, since the donor was drugged and ill.

"When we finally decided to go ahead, the opposition within the hospital began clamoring all over again. Even the cardiologist, who had earlier agreed, stood outside the surgery doors wringing his hands and saying, 'I don't know, I just don't know.' I said, 'Look, when you're going to jump, you're going to jump.' I realized that once this enormous psychological hurdle was cleared, then the others would be easier. We put in the chimp's heart and it started up right away. It beat regularly for a while, but it lasted only two hours because the patient was in terminal shock. He was too sick to accept anything.

"The commotion afterwards was enormous, from the hospital to the pulpits, so we stopped doing them until the immunosuppressive field improved and until we could get better recipients."

Hardy had finished his story. He looked at his watch and excused himself. One more question.

"Had you ever heard of Christiaan Barnard?"

"No. Didn't know the man. Perhaps I had seen his name quite vaguely on some paper about valves. Otherwise, no."

Vincenza, the tiny Italian woman with the reddened, sunken cheeks, developed pneumonia, which dragged on for three weeks, and then she died. It turned out that Leachman had predicted just that; he had, in fact, strongly recommended against her surgery for Ebstein's Disease. An associate, Greek cardiologist Dennis Cokkinos, had argued against him. "When the surgeon is not very good," Cokkinos had said, "then I would vote to wait. But with Cooley and his hands, the cardiologist can afford to be liberal. The girl weighed 78 pounds, she has no life. If we send her back to Italy, do you think she could ever make the trip to Houston again?"

Maria Celestina, the "Please help me" patient, soon thereafter developed a hemothorax—bleeding within the chest cavity—where Cooley had excised the huge aneurysm and replaced it with Dacron. She was rushed back in one night for emergency surgery but Zaorski said there was little hope. "The surgeons in Italy screwed her up royally. Cooley tried to sew stitches into tissue that was like an egg shell."

So many hopeful, hopeless foreigners! The publicity that first DeBakey, and later Cooley, so adroitly courted, coupled with the referrals wooed by hundreds of scholarly papers and lectures and warm welcomes for visiting doctors, had produced a never-ending pilgrimage. Houston was the new Lourdes and the new saints were the old maestro and his banished protégé. "But their families can honestly say to themselves," observed Leachman when he learned of Vincenza's death, "that if the great Doctor Cooley—or DeBakey—could not save their loved one's life, then nobody could. They would much rather think that than have the patient die at home. Then they would cry for the rest of their lives, 'If *only* we had gone to Houston.' "

Cooley had a run on desperately sick Greeks all spring and summer. So many flew to Houston on stretchers, so many were carried into the hospital frothing at the mouth with pulmonary edema, so many died in the hall or on the table or in Recovery, so many should never have left Athens, that Cooley remarked with near melancholy —a remark picked up by several others who started using the line more wryly—"We get so many dying Greeks that they should bring an urn with them when they come to Houston."

On a Friday morning, a fresh death certificate was on the catch-all shelf outside Cooley's surgery office. A youngish Greek fellow in his thirties had died in Intensive Care the night before. Shafi was on duty and when the patient went into left ventricular failure, he could not be resuscitated. The blame for the deaths, Shafi was saying to Bruno Messmer, should be placed with cardiologists who treat patients with operable defects for twenty years. "They wait until the fellow turns blue before they pack him off to Houston."

Dennis Cokkinos, listening to the conversation, said there were several capable cardiovascular surgeons in Athens but that little heart work was being done.

"Why not?" said Jerry Strong. "You've got a pump, don't you?"

"Yes. But they don't operate."

"If you've got balls, use them." Strong was on his way to Room 1, where still another sick Greek, a woman named Anna Zaranikos, was to have two valves replaced.

"They've tried and had some bad results," answered Cokkinos. "Two or three patients died and now nobody will go near the surgeons."

"You've got to educate the people. Hire a press agent, for Christ's sake, and get him to teach people what *can* be done, not what can't."

Nine days after surgery, Vic Coleman, thinner, but cheerful despite his pain and pallor, walked happily out of the hospital. When he returned a week later for a checkup with a new haircut, a new blazer and some beach tan, he hardly looked like a man whose heart had been stopped and altered two weeks before. The incision on his leg, where the vein had been removed, was slightly inflamed with a pus pocket, but Leachman said the skin would flake off shortly and stop the infection.

"Ten days after the operation I walked four-tenths of a mile," Coleman said. "And I'm just about ready to start jogging."

Leachman normally lets patients set their own pace of living, but this seemed to be a man who needed a word of caution. "I'd take it a little bit easy for a couple of months," he said. "It normally takes that long for any major injury to the body to heal, and surgery is a big injury."

"Why did Cooley only do one bypass graft when two had been suggested?"

Leachman, being from Amarillo in the Texas Panhandle and the proud proprietor of a ranch outside Houston where he bred cattle, often used farmer talk for his medical analogies. "Circulation of the heart is rather like irrigation ditches in a corn patch. You might get two or three of them blocked off, but a third would be strong enough to take over and wet the field."

Coleman nodded. What about diet? he wanted to know.

"Well, I wouldn't eat eggs twice a day or meat twice a day, and not too much greasy foods, but aside from that, anything you want."

Coleman looked for Cooley to say thanks and good-bye, but he was in surgery and unavailable.

A patient at Fondren-Brown required emergency surgery a few nights later and George Noon looked for someone to first-assist him. DeBakey was out of town apparently, although his associates rarely knew for sure unless it was an extended overseas trip, a national medical meeting, or an appearance on a network talk show where he could be seen. Ted Diethrich was in Phoenix looking in on Bill Carroll, now completely recovered from his bar crawl. In urgent need of a pair of hands, George called Geoff, the expelled resident, and asked him to scrub. Geoff readily agreed and the operation had been underway but a few moments when the doors to the operating room swung open and there stood DeBakey.

His face a mask of fury, he ordered Geoff to clear out and stay out.

CHAPTER

9

In the quarter of a century since DeBakey had come to Houston, the list of young doctors banished from his surgery was always growing. A few weeks before Geoff's experience, DeBakey had been watching with obvious annoyance the performance of an Italian surgeon who was spending a year in Houston. During an operation, DeBakey instructed the man, whose name was Mario, to sew up the chest incision while he attended to a matter of the femoral artery. When DeBakey was done, he looked up, peered at Mario's sutures, frowned, took his scalpel, and brusquely cut each of them out—replacing them himself, muttering all the while, "If you can't learn, you can't be taught." Later he blew up at Mario and ordered the Italian to "stay out of my sight—I don't even want to *see* you." Mario interpreted this, with help, as meaning that he could not scrub in on DeBakey's service. So he spent the remaining months in Houston assisting the other heart surgeons and slinking about the corridors, hoping he would not encounter DeBakey.

A general surgeon from St. Louis, a patrician-looking doctor with erect posture and gray sideburns to mark his 58 years, gave up his practice and convinced his wife and family that he should go to Houston and spend a year starting over again to learn heart surgery. He made it through the year, but not without frequent crises. During one operation he asked DeBakey a question and the response was several stormy minutes of criticism for having asked it. "You know, Doctor," said DeBakey, witheringly, "by the very nature of your question I wonder if you understand the simple hemodynamics of this case."

DeBakey seemed patient, even kind with the students who came to his table; normally only the man well along in his residency, or his career, felt the heat. "By the time you get to be seniors," he once told a group of freshmen medical students, "we'll be competitors. Don't forget it."

Geoff's sentence was unusually severe. DeBakey had ordered him not only out of the operating room, but also out of the hospital, which meant that he could not finish his year on someone else's service. For days he searched his past conduct and his soul for a reason; the one given by DeBakey hardly seemed to fit the crime, if indeed, in Geoff's opinion, that had been a crime at all. "The final breakup had been coming for three days," Geoff reflected. "Everybody had warned me to watch out. We had already sewed up the patient and we were suturing the wound where a catheter had been stuck into an artery. I was doing nothing but holding the sutures while he cut them, but he said *I* was cutting them off too long. Suddenly he began telling me to get out of the room."

Geoff had come to Houston from New England in 1963 after making applications for residencies at several hospitals around the country. "I hadn't really expected to be chosen for a DeBakey residency. But in typical DeBakey fashion he sent me a telegram saying I had been accepted and to please answer within 24 hours. In other words, I had to commit to four years in Houston within 24 hours. I called friends around the country inquiring about him, and I got all the terror stories about Big Mike. I figured they couldn't be that bad. . . . I was wrong. They were worse.

"I chose Houston because it seemed ideal to be on the frontiers of heart surgery. At other hospitals there might have been one open-heart case a month and 30 residents would be scrubbed in trying to watch. Where else in the world was there a Denton Cooley doing three or four pumps a day? And a George Morris and a Stanley Crawford and all the other heart surgeons turned out by DeBakey?"

Geoff had spent his first year in the Baylor program without being introduced to DeBakey. "He didn't even nod at me in the operating room. Every time a patient died in the Intensive Care Unit, he'd usually fire a guy and blame him for the death. But I also noticed it was usually premeditated. Word would get out that he was after somebody and he'd rag them and pick on them and finally erupt with an enormous harangue and fire them—always in front of everybody. Sometimes these were doctors who needed firing, and always the lesson soaked in. Each time he fired someone, the reason—the alleged reason, because it was not necessarily the real reason—was cemented into all of our brains."

There were DeBakey "quirks" that every resident quickly learned to tolerate and obey. One Geoff learned was his insistence that suture needles be thrown onto the operating room floor after their use. "At other hospitals they don't do that, because the wheels of the stretcher pick them up," Geoff said. "But you damn well learned to throw them on the floor in Mike's room."

Another concerned the surgical drapes. "They must be taut; this is a fetish, little else."

A third, and cardinal, rule related to the lights. DeBakey uses four overhead, movable, sterile spots. Most surgeons (Cooley, for example) use only two. "The unwritten, unspoken, but religiously observed law is that the light opposite the Professor does not shine onto the field, because it bounces off the retractors and annoys him. If anybody dares to touch those lights. . . ."

But Geoff had not touched the lights nor broken the other rules. He had stayed seven years learning his craft and was on the threshhold of his surgical majority when the blade fell. Perhaps one thing he had done to annoy DeBakey was to admire Denton Cooley's skill —Cooley, after all, *had* been a member of the Baylor surgical faculty until a few months before—and he had gone to an occasional party with Cooley's fellows. But if those were contributing factors, Geoff could no more understand it than he could understand DeBakey. And after seven years, he had found no Rosetta Stone to help him. "He has taught me virtually nothing, because we had hardly a relationship at all. But the years were valuable, nonetheless.

The things Mike had taught the others, and the improvements they had added, these things seeped down to me. Everything emanates from Mike! Suture technique, for example, which is the basis for all vascular work, was developed by Mike. Invented? No, developed. But what is 'invented' anyway? Some dodo off in the North Woods might have done the first abdominal aneurysm, but unless he was shrewd enough to market it and run with it and publish it—who knew? Who cared?"

And that, certainly, was something he learned from Mike De-Bakey.

DeBakey! Ask six doctors to describe him and they become six blind men telling of the elephant. Don Bricker says there is "the charming DeBakey, the tyrannical DeBakey, the gracious DeBakey, the political DeBakey, the despot DeBakey, and original healer DeBakey."

In his ninth and last year in Houston, Don Bricker held one of the most important positions in the Baylor program—he ran the vast surgery service at Ben Taub General, the huge charity hospital that served America's sixth largest city. DeBakey actually held the title of "Surgeon-in-Chief" at Ben Taub, but on his priority of participation, it was well down the line, so far down as to be practically non-existent. Bricker relished the responsibility and wide pathology of the Taub job, but he gave notice in mid-1970 that he was quitting to go to Lubbock, a growing town in West Texas, where he would start up a private heart-surgery service from scratch.

Bricker's reasoning pointed up both the nature and the dilemma of the modern surgeon. Surgery, until quite recently, was a specialty of medicine in itself. "Suddenly," said Bricker, "we are in the era of the super-specialist, the super-surgeon, and the only way to get ahead in my racket is to do one thing better than anybody else. I have the widest repertoire of any surgeon in Houston—at the age of 35—but I'm a dinosaur. I don't specialize. I've decided to go to a place where I can."

In every aspect but one, Bricker's appearance and dossier matched the classic image of the young Houston heart surgeon. He had a strong, open face; a compact, well-controlled body (DeBakey once snapped at an overweight resident, " I never knew a good fat doctor, Doctor!"), his clothes were quiet and from the rack of an Ivy League shop, his politics were conservative, his wife was a former nurse, his nonmedical passion was sports and the souping up of ordinary cars, and he swam in his pool with his three sons and a giant black dog, who was the most able water-polo player in the household. Only his attitude regarding his moral responsibility as surgeon toward the patient differed from what I had grown familiar with. Scattered among the gunshot wounds, the radical breasts, the crushed chests were but a few open-heart cases a month. But for each of these —charity bum, junkie, hooker, or forgotten old man—he not only repaired the heart, but went afterward into the Recovery Room and put a blanket on the floor and slept beside the bed. "I think it is necessary that I stay beside my patient until he has no further need of the surgeon," he said, cutting off further conversation on the subject as men do when elaboration on a deeply held belief seems unnecessary.

Bricker had come to Houston in 1961 from New York Hospital, where he had become enamored of the then still infant area of open-heart surgery. "But there was nobody in New York to teach it, so I applied to DeBakey. He asked me but one question, was I a member of Alpha Omega Alpha, the medical honor fraternity. I said yes, and I was hired."

His residency was more tempestuous than most. "When it was done, if I had to choose between going back to DeBakey's service for three months or going to Vietnam to do battlefield surgery for three months, I'd choose Vietnam. Now that it is over, I have tremendous respect and affection for the man, but there were days when I wanted to kill him. I'd stand there and let him punch me on the chest with his stabbing fingers and listen to his tirades and I'd have my fists clenched behind my back."

On other days DeBakey would be harassing someone and Bricker noticed that the deeply browed eyes were sparkling during the tirade. "I think he's actually having fun doing this," thought Bricker at the time.

During the decade of the 1960s, the widely held opinion in the surgical world was that DeBakey, although an excellent surgeon, was not as technically gifted as Cooley. Bricker had stood across the

table from both men during hundreds of operations and had come
to conclusions on both men's abilities:

"Cooley had and has a particular genius for taking the bits and
pieces of another doctor's work, then putting it together again in a
new whole to suit himself—and doing it better than anybody in the
world. He has advanced heart surgery more than any other man.
I'm not as good as Denton in the operating room; nobody could be
until he's done 6,000 hearts—and then you still wouldn't be Denton
Cooley.

"But DeBakey's surgery was also a thing of astonishing beauty.
He, too, was an incredible technician, but it was, for those assisting,
a very traumatic episode."

By 1965, Bricker's fourth year of residency, DeBakey was enjoying the fallout from two public relation coups—his appearance on
the cover of *Time* magazine and his operation on the Duke of Windsor for an abdominal aneurysm—which increased his patient census
to as many as 200 at one time, enough to fill an entire respectable-
sized hospital. "And the Professor expected his resident to know
literally everything about every patient. He'd chew you out for
something you had absolutely no control over. He never quits, he
persists beyond reason.

"Once he ripped into me for the hundredth time over something
and I was ready to tell him off and get out. At that moment somebody came up and told me I was wanted down at Admitting because
there was some hassle over a Spanish-speaking family. I speak Spanish and I went down and encountered a ragtag-looking couple from
Bolivia and their sick kid. All they had was a cardboard suitcase and
a crumpled yellow telegram. I read it, and it said 'If you will come
to Houston on such and such a date, I will operate for no fee on
your child. Signed, Michael DeBakey, M.D.' I melted. DeBakey in all
his power had reached out to a Bolivian village and touched this
poor, pathetic family."

During his DeBakey years, Bricker watched several of his col-
leagues thrown off the service. "I finally came to believe that nobody
got fired who didn't need firing. DeBakey is celebrated for axing people on a whim, but it was usually a whim he had invented as an
excuse, a last straw, because he had watched them and had been
ready to fire them for weeks. Some teachers give you questions to

answer, DeBakey puts you under this enormous stress, he pushes you as far as you will go, sometimes beyond human reason, and if you can't take it, you're out."

The strain on the younger doctors was not wholly mental; often their bodies would collapse and they would fall ill, but because De-Bakey did not tolerate personal illness, he did not expect his residents to get sick either. (For a man of 62, DeBakey takes dismal care of himself. I once asked him when was the last time *he* had had an EKG, since he spends every day reading those of others. "I can't remember," he said, almost sheepishly. "Have you *ever* had one?" I pressed. He shook his head negatively. His personal nutrition would distress the mother of any adolescent. All day long he snacks on chocolate candy and peanuts and caramel-covered popcorn. Once when we dined at a fashionable New York steak house he ordered a strip sirloin and when it came, impeccably cooked, he asked for a bottle of Tabasco sauce, the fiery concoction two drops of which can ignite a Bloody Mary. Taking the bottle he slathered his steak with Tabasco, spreading it from end to end as one would spread tomato sauce over a veal cutlet. His fondness for Tabasco, a product of his native Louisiana, caused one associate to say, "Mike DeBakey puts Tabasco on everything he eats—and everything he says.")

Once, Bricker recalled, DeBakey turned up in the operating room with a terrible cold, made even more insufferable by the mask over his mouth and nose. "He sniffled around and growled like a lion with a sore paw. I slipped out and went down to the pharmacy and got him a bag full of antibiotics and antihistamines and rather boldly thrust it on him and told him to take it. He poked around the bag and said, 'This stuff's no good; the only thing that works is aspirin.' I insisted that he go home early—like 8 P.M. instead of midnight—and take some. The next morning he was obviously better. He sidled up to me and said, 'Do you think you could get me some more of that stuff?' "

On another day, DeBakey was felled with a severe virus but he insisted on going to surgery. He was, said Bricker, "so pale, so sick, that the team almost forcibly made him lie down on the OR table. He was vomiting and feverish and furious. Someone notified the chairman of the department of medicine, who came down and took one look at Mike and ordered him to take the day off and rest. Mike refused to leave the hospital. 'Very well,' said the chairman, 'you can have a room in the hospital, but if we have to tie you up and take you there, we will.' Complaining bitterly, Mike got off the table, bolted out of the OR, ran up four flights of stairs to prove that—even sick—he was a better man than anybody else, lay down on a hospital bed and slept eight hours straight through. As much as we hated him, we were sad that the lion was sick. He was back the next day yelling at us. So we knew he felt better."

There came the day when Bricker almost threw away his medical career. He had advanced to chief resident, an exalted position in other surgical training programs but under DeBakey still very much a junior man. A 25-year-old patient in the Intensive Care Unit who had been operated on for repair of a ventricular septal defect suddenly developed a hemothorax in his left chest and was bleeding to death. Bricker almost tore open his chest and sucked blood out and got it under control, then ran into surgery and told DeBakey the patient would have to come back in for emergency repair.

"DeBakey was furious," remembered Bricker. "He always was when the schedule was interrupted, but he agreed to let me bring the boy in. For two hours he stood over me and yelled that the mistake should have been caught the night before and repaired then. He gave me unmerciful hell. The boy had had his VSD operation that *very morning*, not the day before, and DeBakey had done it, not me. Finally I had all I could take. I stripped off my gloves, I broke scrub, I lunged across the table for the Professor and tried to get my hands around his throat. Ed Garrett and Jimmy Howell grabbed me and physically dragged me out of the OR. I went back to ICU and kicked the wall."

Bricker hung low for three days, assuming that he would be kicked far out of not only Methodist, but out of medicine as well. On the fourth dark day, word was sent that DeBakey wanted Bricker present at a staff conference. "I went in scared to death, but ready to take whatever he was going to dish out. I was surprised to find that it was an ordinary patient conference. DeBakey was looking at some x-rays and he turned to me and said, 'Don, I just don't know what to do for this patient. What do you suggest?'"

It was DeBakey's business-as-usual way of acknowledging a mistake and inviting Bricker back into the program.

In August of 1970, Bricker went to the Cooley camp and filled in for Grady Hallman while he was on holiday. Although now a grown-up surgeon, very much his own man, so to speak, and on his way to Lubbock and private practice, he worked the entire two weeks almost furtively, worried that DeBakey would hear of his favor and pronounce him disloyal.

During the period, Bricker overheard a coffee-room conversation between two fellows who were complaining that they were not allowed to do any actual heart surgery under Cooley. In the entire year, they would do nothing but assist and tend to the patients before and after. They had come expecting to actually get their hands into hearts—with Cooley standing beside them giving advice and counsel.

"I know how they feel," Bricker said later, on a Sunday afternoon beside his pool, watching the big black dog chase his sons in the churning water. "What can you learn watching Cooley do a thousand patients? There is nothing so frightening, nothing so gut-wrenching as the moment when someone finally hands you a knife and says—'Here, cut this heart.'"

"For more than a year now, I've been all pent up," said Ted Diethrich on another steamy new summer Sunday afternoon. "I haven't made a contribution in twelve months, except banging out these hearts day after day." He was sitting on the patio of his splendid, low-slung brick home in suburban Houston, an old house rebuilt to his specifications for embracing the outdoors. Walls of glass slide open for instant access to the large pool. There is a curious-looking athletic court—the only one in the United States—with three cathedral-like brick walls for the playing of a passionate and violent form of Mexican sport called frontenis. There is an adjoining vacant lot for football. Every Sunday, after morning hospital rounds, Diethrich would lead a pack of young heart surgeons and medical students through an orgy of athletic endeavor which, well-fueled by vodka and tonic, would stretch deep into the night. It became a pursuit of the fine edge of complete exhaustion, a search for physical pain, the cleansing purge that would send the surgeon back to the hospital and its world of imperfect minds and bodies.

On occasional Sundays, Diethrich asked an important, recuperating patient out to his home, and the man, still feeble from surgery, would sit in a chair with his shirt unbuttoned. He would watch the handsome, strong, young men pummeling each other at water polo, hear their shouting on the tennis court, feel the spray as they tossed themselves into the pool. No doubt the man was happy to leave the hospital for an hour or two, even with the nurse and her blood pressure cuff beside him, but as he watched the spectacle, there came a sadness, which only I saw, in his eyes.

Sundays tore at me. I recognized the need to push out the traumas of the week, but I would have preferred to accomplish it on a 30-15 ratio—30 minutes of sport, 15 minutes of chair. The surgeon syndrome had different rules, more like 58 and 2. Frontenis was undeniably exhilarating, entwining elements of handball, jai alai, and tennis, but with the hard rubber ball hurtling past at speeds up to 80 miles per hour, it was alarming as well. By the end of the summer, my torso, as were those of the other players, was dotted with bruises. My elbow was blue-green and swollen. "If you're going to have a heart attack," one of the doctors said cheerfully, "this is not a bad place to have one."

Earlier in the year I had skied with Diethrich and a group of Michigan surgeons in Aspen. The other men were all ten years our senior but they seemed to have taken the same oath as Diethrich. I am a skier and I love the sport but my notion is to tear off a thousand-yard descent or so, stop, find a chalet with hot wine, and look at the trees. Not the surgeons. Their idea of skiing was to rise at dawn and be first in the lift line—very important, being first—be first to the top of the mountain, be first to the bottom of the mountain, over and over again, until threatening shadows threw fingers across the runs. No stopping. No reflecting. No wasted moment.

Among surgeons who fly their own airplanes—and there are many —the rate of crash and death is *four times* that of the businessman pilot. One reason is the surgeon's rush to return to the hospital on Monday morning. Another, I suspect, is the surgeon's desperate bear hug on life, paired with the feeling—as some Las Vegas gamblers have—that God sits on their shoulder and will not allow His blessed ones to lose.

At the age of 35, Diethrich had reached a level of professional reputation and personal reward that other surgeons would not reach until their fifth or sixth decade. But as it had with so many before him, a restlessness was setting in. The pattern was well established. If the young doctor survived the residency program and if he was exceptionally skilled in the operating room, DeBakey would ask him to stay on in the Baylor program. He would receive an academic appointment to the surgical faculty and he would assist De-Bakey on his cases. He would also be permitted to establish his own private practice, keeping a small percentage of his fees. The balance went to the medical college; DeBakey turned over between 50 and 75 percent of his to the department.

But how many men have sat close to the throne without wondering if the chair is comfortable? The doctor who relaxed in the St. Luke's coffee room one midnight and figured on his scrub suit leg the potential income of Denton Cooley had not been the first man to multiply the staggering figures. And the 27-story tower of St. Luke's hospital, of which Cooley's Texas Heart Institute would occupy a considerable section, dominated the Texas Medical Center as the Shell Building did downtown Houston. Cooley's hands had built one hospital; DeBakey's hands—and power—had built another. It had not escaped Diethrich's attention, and he was even then nursing a plan.

Diethrich was born in Michigan. His mother was a nurse and he did his first operations on stuffed animals when he was five. He was in the hospital working as an orderly by the time he was fourteen. At fifteen he assisted and actually did the cutting on a vasectomy—male sterilization—and he could never remember a time when he was not consumed with ambition to be a surgeon. There had been a period when he pointed himself toward neurosurgery, that last glamour specialty, but by the time he had completed his surgical residency at the University of Michigan, he had been converted to a future in the heart. He applied to several hospitals for the necessary two-year thoracic-surgery residence but held little hope that he could be accepted by DeBakey. The University of Michigan had and has one of the most respected thoracic programs in the world of medicine but it required equal surgical time all over the chest cavity; Diethrich knew Houston concentrated on the heart.

"Finally a letter came from Baylor saying I had been accepted and I went down to Houston to meet DeBakey. I waited hours, I sat outside his office, I watched him operate, I followed him up and down stairs. Finally at five in the afternoon, after he had finished doing a beautiful arch aneurysm on a captain in the Air Force, he walked up to me and spoke to me for perhaps 30 seconds. He said 'Very glad to have you here; I hope we see you soon.' I was struck stone dead. I was in the presence of God."

On July 1, the traditional end and beginning of the medical year, 1964, Diethrich presented himself to DeBakey's office and much to his surprise was assigned to Denton Cooley. Cooley already had become estranged from Mike DeBakey and had shifted his surgery to neighboring St. Luke's. But Cooley at that time was still very much a member of the Baylor surgical faculty—indeed he contributed half of his enormous surgical fees to the department of surgery—and he was entitled to a resident. Diethrich became disenchanted very quickly. Accustomed to the academic, ordered scheme at Michigan, he was confused by the breakneck atmosphere of Houston medicine. "I was used to a program where someone said, 'This is who you are, Doctor, this is what you do, this is where you can progress to.' Instead, it seemed to be a jumble. There were about 40,000 people jammed into the operating room, you couldn't even get near Cooley. I was totally lost the first month."

When he rotated several months later onto DeBakey's service, Diethrich found himself even further from the operating room. For two and one half months he was not even invited into surgery, this young doctor who had just completed four years at Michigan operating almost every day. One afternoon, DeBakey abruptly said, "Ted, you've got to develop yourself technically in the operating room—starting tomorrow, I want you to scrub in with me on every single case." Diethrich bit his tongue to keep from saying that judgment on his need for technical development seemed premature, since DeBakey had never seen him tie a single knot.

"Well, we started that," recalls Diethrich. "The first three or four days went perfectly. He didn't say anything to me, all was quiet, it was going to be everything I had hoped it would be. I was in the presence of the master. Then came the months of hell. It was to be the worst experience of my whole life. It got so bad he wouldn't even let me drape the patient, something I had been doing for years, as routinely as reading a thermometer. I hold the all-time record for draping a patient! It was a carotid operation (reaming out the artery in the neck to prevent strokes) and I got the patient ready and De-Bakey came in and took one look and said it was not properly done. So he went out and I took the drapes off and opened another sterile package and draped the patient again. DeBakey came the second time and again it was wrong. So I took the drapes off and broke open a new package and did it again. And again! And again! Four drapings! It got so bad I couldn't tie a knot in the operating room without doing it wrong. It got so bad the anesthesiologist said to me one day, 'Ted, I just dread to see you come into this operation room.'

"I never made it through a case with him. I'd make the incision wrong. I couldn't hold a retractor. I was standing in the light. Everything was wrong. He'd say, 'Why can't you do this for me, Doctor, why, why, WHY? Don't you *want* to help me, Doctor? This doctor doesn't *want* to help me!'

"We'd start a case, we'd get about ten minutes into it, he'd stop and throw up his hands and say, 'Ted, would you get Dr. Garrett?' Somebody would go and get Dr. Garrett and DeBakey would banish me to a corner and say, 'You just stand over there, Doctor.'

"It got to a point where I lost all my confidence. He can shatter you, absolutely shatter you. He would say to the whole operating room, 'It must be *intentional*—nobody could operate like this unless it was intentional.' I never answered back to him. I never raised my voice, because this was what provoked him the most. It went on day after day after day until one afternoon he laid down the instruments and he said, 'All right, Doctor, all right. This is it. *This is it!* You obviously do not want to assist me. You want to be number one. Doctor, *I'm* going to assist *you*. Here, you take this forceps, and you take this needle, and you take this suture, and *you* sew up the artery.' I started in and it lasted about 30 seconds before he grabbed everything back from me."

The harangue dragged on until Diethrich fell into depression. He would return home late at night and tell his wife, Gloria, "This man is intentionally trying to break me. It's become a battle." There were days when Diethrich would put on his scrubs and then fight down nausea at the thought of going into surgery. He would go to Ed Garrett, a surgeon who had been through the ordeal and who was now a member of the Baylor faculty and ask for help. "Ed, I don't know how much more of this I can take. I'm losing my confidence, I dread to walk into the operating room, and I've loved the operating room since I was fifteen." He went to Jimmy Howell, another surgeon, and begged him to scrub in and take his place and Howell would say, "I don't even want to be near it."

"I was a person who had devoted so many years to becoming technically proficient, to achieving a certain skill, and to be ground down under his heel was frightening," Diethrich said.

After three months, DeBakey approached Diethrich in the hallway early one morning and said, hurriedly, "You take Room 4 today." Diethrich's knees almost buckled. This meant he would be operating alone, with a junior man assisting *him*. "From that moment on, it was night suddenly day. He respected my judgment. He'd come in and assist me, or I'd go in and assist him and nothing more was said."

Diethrich never knew what he had done to pass the test because he never understood the rules of the test. Or even if there was a test. Or why DeBakey chose and chose again to seize the Roman candle of youth and shake it and press his hands down on it and snuff out the fires of desire and ambition until the sparks—sodden with tears and sweat—were all but gone. Reporters sometimes asked DeBakey how he dealt with death and he usually replied with a reference to Irving Stone's novel of Michelangelo, but he invariably mixed up the title. "It is the Ecstasy and the Agony for we heart surgeons," he said. "To win is ecstasy, to lose is agony." But was his vision of the business so painful that he chose to sort out those he would permit to enter?

Diethrich had come to believe that only those doctors from outside the Baylor program fell victim to DeBakey's ire. One night as DeBakey and Diethrich drove to the Methodist Annex and were talking of a resident to whom the senior surgeon had been giving holy hell, DeBakey suddenly stopped and was silent for a while. His hands were on the steering wheel and he clutched it tightly. He began to speak again in a flat, cold voice. "Ted," he said, "you know, I test people. I see what people can do under fire and under pressure. I *must* know what these people are made of."

I dined at the home of a college friend who was now a successful surgeon and who had been through the DeBakey program. How alike the memoirs were becoming! I could almost recite along with him. "He put me through hell's fire," said my friend, whose face grew tight as he remembered it. "He used to say, 'You are so stupid, you must be mentally retarded. Mentally retarded: Anyone who acts like you do must have brain damage. We're going to take you right into surgery and fix your carotid artery. I don't think we even need an arteriogram.' He used to stand me up against the corner and jab those fingers of his into my chest and it was like being stabbed."

His hand went to his shirt and he searched for an imaginary cavity.

"But now it's over," I said. "What do you think of the man?"

"Oh," he began quickly, "I. . . ." He stopped. He had formed the syllable "L" with his lips but the word, that automatic word, that easiest word, would not come. "I . . . *like* him, I respect him," my friend said. "He gave me opportunities that nobody else would have. He also built up Baylor in twenty years to where it ranked with Harvard and Johns Hopkins and it took those schools 200 years to get there."

My friend stopped. He measured what he would say. "But he cannot run Baylor and be a full-time practicing surgeon . . . *and* fight the world. . . . How lonely he must be."

On the next Sunday afternoon the green phone on the table beside Diethrich's pool rang and he stopped playing tennis to take the call. It was from the hospital.

"Who was it?" one of the surgeons asked.

"Howard Stapler just checked back in in heart failure."

"What can you do for him?" I asked.

"Transplant him, I guess," said Diethrich, and he picked up the ball to serve.

PART TWO

The Transplant Era

"... there ensued what appeared to be an international race to be a member of the me-too brigade. There has not been anything like it in medical annals. ..."

— Dr. Irvine Page, cardiologist, 1968 winner of the American Medical Association's award as the country's "Outstanding Physician."

C H A P T E R
10

One day in the early 1960s at a Saturday morning patient conference at St. Luke's Hospital there arose the problem of a man whose heart was so deteriorated that it could not tolerate Cooley's surgery. Otherwise his body was youthful and strong. When all the hopeless avenues of potential treatments had been traveled, someone from the back of the conference room called out, "Transplant him!"

Transplant him! Sew in a new heart! But where would that heart come from? Someone else would have to *die* in order to contribute that borrowed heart. "I have an idea," one of the younger doctors said. "Why not move the patient *and* the operating room to Huntsville?" Huntsville, 75 miles north of Houston, is the site of Texas' huge central prison and home of its once-active electric chair. "We could obtain permission from a condemned murderer to use his heart," the young doctor theorized, "and the night they executed him, we'd be there to take out his heart and transplant it into our man. . . ."

Nothing came of the bizarre scheme, but the imaginative doctor was not totally hooted down. Talk of transplants peppered American medicine as the decade of the 1960s began. There was scarcely a medical center without at least one transplant research project, if not swapping hearts and lungs and kidneys and spleens and bone marrow and endocrine tissue in dogs and calves, then at least in hamsters or mice. In Mississippi, Dr. James Hardy transplanted the ovaries and uterus *en bloc* from ten female dogs to ten recipients. Three of the ten not only tolerated the new organs, they later became pregnant and gave birth to healthy litters. In Denver, Dr. Tom Starzl led a team that was slowly moving kidney transplantation out of the realm of rare, audacious surgery—greatly discouraging at first and applicable only in giving a kidney taken from one identical twin to another—onward to where more than 10,000 kidneys would be taken from cadaver donors and implanted in recipients. The kidney transplant would become, in the 1960s, a majestic and routine piece of surgery performed all over America.

But what of the heart? And the brain? The transplanted brain, as far as the state of medical knowledge and expertise extended, was out of the question. Nervous tissue is not regenerative; it would not grow in another system.* The heart was clearly the jackpot of transplantation surgery, and many American surgeons moved in the early 1960s to claim it. At Stanford University, Dr. Norman Shumway and Dr. Richard Lower began a series of transplanting hundreds of dog hearts, refining and polishing their surgical technique that would later become the basis for all heart transplantation. At the University of Mississippi, Dr. Hardy moved toward his historic chimpanzee heart-into-man operation in 1963. And in Houston, Mike DeBakey chose to go for a heart that would not be wrapped in legal, moral, and probably religious brambles. Shrewdly, DeBakey decided to let the others test their hearts from dogs, chimps, and cadavers. *His* would be plastic and metal. He would build and implant an *artificial* heart. There was little doubt in his mind that it could be done. He had already pioneered and made common the implantation of plastic patches into veins and arteries, of artificial valves into hearts. It would be the astonishing climax to an astonishing career.

---

* *Not totally out of the realm of possibility is that entire heads might be transplanted some decade hence. Russian surgeons grafted the head of a dog onto another in 1954, and the animal lived briefly. If an entire human head were transplanted, the donor would, in effect, become the recipient, because his brain would be transferred to another body.*

Such an undertaking would require a large sum of money. De-Bakey went after it. Always a clever player of the academic game called "grantsmanship," he had commuted with regularity to the centers of power and money in America—Washington and New York. And he had cultivated important friends—Mary Lasker of the rich and prestigious Lasker Medical Foundation, cardiologist Paul Dudley White, certain congressmen. "Mike does not go to parties unless there is at least a congressman present," observed a DeBakey watcher, "and preferably that congressman is the chairman of an appropriations committee." Careful sifting of his invitations and of those who would become his friend paid well. Over the years De-Bakey personally raised more than $50 million for his projects, and, in 1962, pulled out a plum that any medical center in America would have relished: a $2.5 million grant to devise and develop an artificial heart. Quickly he moved to spend it and the millions that would follow. He set up laboratories at Baylor, bought equipment, scouted for people. One he hired was a talented and ambitious Argentine surgeon named Domingo Liotta, a quiet, handsome Latin who spoke English with difficulty but whose mind seemed geared toward the painstaking work of building and discarding scores of models, of experimenting with plastics and rubber and velour, of huddling with engineers to perfect the best possible power source to drive the man-made pump.

A Baylor faculty member described the scene. "DeBakey was ecstatic. He had always adored his hours in the laboratory, tinkering with plastic and metal and pliers and scissors. He would have made a great engineer had he not turned to medicine. His zeal, his enthusiasm inspired everyone. He made each feel that the goal was the most important scientific contribution of our time. It would surpass Curie, it would surpass Einstein. . . ."

Not surprisingly, the press discovered DeBakey.

Scientists have traditionally shied away from the flashbulb; De-Bakey welcomed cameras and notebooks into his cloistered world. In 1963 he agreed to perform a heart-valve operation on the first live worldwide satellite television broadcast via Early Bird. The carefully scripted program opened with mariachis (Mexican street bands) playing in Mexico City, thence to an oom-pah-pah concert in Essen, Germany, and on to Operating Room 4 at the Methodist Hospital

of Houston, where TV cameras, placed and rehearsed by Michael De-
Bakey, were actually within the surgical suite, two scuttling side-
ways across the tiled walls, a third in the glass dome for overhead
angles. "Now here is where you zoom down, at just about eleven
o'clock," said DeBakey in rehearsal to the camerman on high. "Can
you visualize it correctly?" The cameraman nodded. DeBakey hurried about his staff, cautioning his assistants not to get their heads in
the way. Two hundred million people watched DeBakey at his best.

Three years later he permitted a *Life* magazine photographer and
reporter to wait in Houston off and on for almost a year until a suitable patient turned up to receive a left ventricular bypass, half an
artificial heart. Their first attempts at devising an entire pump had
been discouraging, so Liotta and his staff had created the ventricular
bypass and had proved its efficiency in animal tests. In 1966, such an
implantation in a human being was a dramatic and newsworthy piece
of surgery. Although the case that *Life* photographed was not a
happy one—the patient died two days after surgery—the ten-page
color spread firmly established DeBakey as the leading searcher
for an artificial heart. A shower of criticism fell on him from his
peers for his courtship of the press, for his inviting journalists into
the operating room, for his news conferences and television appearances. Characteristically, DeBakey paid small heed to the complaints.
He acted, he said, to inform the public about the progress made with
federal funds—the *people's* money, he emphasized. "The people have
a right to know what we are doing with their tax money," he said.
And if Mike DeBakey became, coincidentally, the most famous surgeon in America, then it was a by-product over which he had no
control.

DeBakey's shadow was so enormous in the period 1960–67 that
Denton Cooley worked in relative darkness. His name appeared on
scores of medical papers adjoining the senior authorship of Mike
DeBakey, and the world of medicine pronounced their names almost
as if a hyphen joined them. But the relationship that had begun as
polite and professional in 1951 became, by 1960, stiff and chilly.
There was never a dramatic break, only a gradual moving away,
an erosion. Cooley simply found it more and more difficult to get
operating-room space for his own cases at Methodist. One member
of the Baylor surgical faculty remembers getting to the hospital be-

fore sunrise and making up imaginary names and procedures and filling them in on the blackboard to reserve space for DeBakey. Cooley
also fretted at the traditional academic custom of the chairman of a
department adding his name to all papers written by the men beneath
him. This is done to facilitate indexing in medical libraries of the
thousands of scientific papers that are written every year, and to
emphasize the responsibility the chairman has for the work that goes
on beneath him.

"Denton felt that every time he did something important," said a
surgeon of that era, "Mike got credit for it. Denton had become the
best heart cutter in the world and nobody outside the medical socie-
ties knew his name." *He'd* certainly never been on television before
200 million people.

Cooley's gifted hands were turning up hundreds of thousands of
dollars in surgical fees for the Baylor department, yet every time he
asked for something—he complained to a friend—be it a piece of
equipment, a resident to assist him, a secretary to handle his records,
"there was a hassle with Mike."

"There were a thousand little things between them," said one observer, "but basically it was the incompatibility of two enormous
egos. Denton flat got tired of sucking hind tit. One day after some
bickering over something—a valve replacement, maybe a coarcta-
tion, I forget which—Denton said in a quiet little voice that hardly
anybody heard, 'Okay, Groucho, have it your way!' Mike had a
mustache then and looked a little like Groucho Marx. And Denton
left and went across the way to St. Luke's and, in effect, never came
back."

When Cooley began working alone at St. Luke's and Texas Children's, it was the first time in his life that he had been without a
dominant male figure. "He was never close to his father, nor was he
close to Mike," said a boyhood friend, "but both were strong,
glamorous over-powering objects. Those of us who knew Denton
figured that he had to see if he could make it as his own man."

On the first day of December, 1967, Dr. James Nora faced the
unpleasant task of telling a young couple that there was nothing
surgically available for their newborn child. The infant had been

delivered with a hypoplastic heart, an unusual condition in which the left side of the heart is underdeveloped, coupled with atresia of two valves. "The only thing to do would be to change hearts," Nora speculated. "Someday it might be feasible, perhaps—someday in the future. If the child can live that long, we could do it."

Twenty-four hours later, a bulletin flashed across the world from Groote Schuur Hospital in Cape Town, South Africa:

> The first human-to-human heart transplant in history was done last night by a team of doctors at the Groote Schuur Hospital. The name of the patient, as well as the donor, are being withheld by hospital authorities.
>
> The heart transplant team was led by Professor Christiaan Barnard in a dramatic all-night operation—the first of its kind in medical history. Messages of congratulation are pouring in from around the world. . . ."

The parents of the doomed baby hurried up to Nora in a corridor of St. Luke's. That far-off "someday" had arrived with breathtaking suddenness. Could Cooley transplant the heart of someone else into their baby? "I don't know," said Nora, surprised as was everyone else in Houston at the Cape Town bulletins. "I'll see." He found Cooley outside surgery. "You want to get into the transplant business?" asked Nora. Cooley nodded his head affirmatively and said, "Sure."

Five months would go by and the child with the hypoplastic heart would die before the transplant era would begin in Cooley's surgery. While surgeons around the world hurried to join the list and the headlines of those who attempted the procedure, Cooley held back. He seemed to have little enthusiasm for transplants. In speeches he publicly congratulated Barnard on the breakthrough, but warned against haste in pronouncing the operation as a cure-all for heart disease.

Three days after Barnard transplanted a heart into Louis Washkansky, Dr. Adrian Kantrowitz became the first American surgeon to attempt—and fail—in the procedure. He installed a new heart in the chest of a newborn child, but the infant died six and a half hours after the operation in Brooklyn's Maimonides Hospital. A month later, in Stanford Medical Center, Dr. Norman Shumway attempted his first; the recipient lived but fifteen days. Shumway's near decade of intense research in transplantation, and the knowledge obtained from swapping hundreds of animal hearts, had made him the pre-eminent figure in the field. One of the ironies of the transplant era was that had Shumway been the first—had the hands of Shumway been the first to lift a heart from a dying body and put it into a living man—then the medical world would have said, in effect, "Of course Shumway did it. He was eminently qualified to do it. He has done more research on the procedure than any man in the world and we have read his papers and heard his speeches and if any man must try it, then Shumway is he. . . ."

But Christiaan Barnard was first, and few had even heard of Christiaan Barnard, and the world was not accustomed to dramatic breakthroughs occurring in South Africa. If a heart transplant could be done by an obscure surgeon at the bottom of the world, then it must not be all that difficult. Barnard, moreover, was blessed with good fortune. His first transplant lived but eighteen days. But his second, the dentist Philip Blaiberg, would live for almost two years.

"As long as Blaiberg was alive," said Bob Leachman in Houston, "he was Columbus setting out for the New World. Until he proved otherwise, we could believe there might be a New World."

Denton Cooley had not actively participated for many years in the Baylor research program. In the decade of the 1950s he had been instrumental in improving and perfecting the heart-lung by-pass machine and in testing the many artificial valves that the labora-tories conceived for use in human hearts. But when he shifted his career to St. Luke's and Texas Children's, he seldom if ever went near the labs. He had, in fact, become skeptical of the value of doing ex-tensive practice heart surgery in dogs. Twelve years earlier, in 1956, he had been pushed—reluctantly—into his first open-heart operation in a human being. A Houston cardiologist, Dr. Sidney Schnurr, had a 58-year-old male patient who had suffered a severe heart attack, followed by a rupture of the septum—creating a perilous hole in the heart. Schnurr urged Cooley to put the man on the then infant and unpredictable bypass pump, stop his heart, and sew up the hole.

"I don't think we're ready yet," Cooley had said.

"This man is going to die," Schnurr replied with passion.

"The dogs have *all* died on the pump. I've done hundreds and they've all died. There are still too many problems."

"To hell with problems," snapped Schnurr. "This is an opportunity for you to do your first human open-heart case."

Cooley walked in meditation around the corridors of the hospital for a quarter of an hour. He paced the halls and stood alone for a time on a stair landing. Finally he returned to Schnurr and said quietly and with apprehension, "Okay."

The man lived but two months and autopsy revealed that the sutures that closed the hole in the heart had pulled out. Cooley's error had been in placing them too close within the necrotic tissue. He learned to sew them farther away in later operations. He also learned that human physiology behaves with considerable difference on the pump than that of the dog.

"Humans will tolerate this surgery much better than dogs," Cooley said years later. "Dogs, for some reason, don't like to have their blood bubbled through the pump oxygenator. And, of course, the dogs we had for experimental purposes in those days were sick animals. They were strays, diseased, they took surgery badly. It was like trying to operate on a human with an acute blood-stream infection." (A famous article appeared in a medical journal of that period entitled "Man's Best Friend?" which said, in effect, that extensive experimental work on dogs had held back human open-heart surgery for at least ten years.)

"Are you going to do any transplants?" asked a Houston newspaper reporter of Cooley at a cocktail party in the early winter of 1968. "We might," he said. "We're looking into it."

"What do you think of them?" asked the reporter.

"Like the man who ate the first oyster," Cooley said, "it took courage."

Christiaan Barnard launched his world tour, a triumphant torero circling the ring, a newly confirmed *celebrity* trailing clippings, television cameras, spotlights, applause, and beautiful women. Cooley attended a medical meeting in South America and found himself swept up in the crowds and sirens and motorcycle escorts for Barnard. Reporters mobbed the corridors of the hotel where the two surgeons were staying. Cooley returned to Houston and recounted the scene, adding, almost sorrowfully, "I went there as a surgeon with the largest cardiac series in the history of medicine, and nobody even knew my name."

By May 1, 1968, eight transplants had been done throughout the world and all save Philip Blaiberg had quickly died. In Bombay, India, a patient lived but three hours with his new heart. In Paris, two days. Shumway's second try lasted but three and a half days. Kantrowitz's second, only eight and a half hours. The survival times seemed mainly to be measured in hours and days—not years or decades. The miracle of Cape Town had turned bleak. But there was still that testy dentist with the heart of a young black beating within him. Blaiberg was giving interviews and signing contracts for his memoirs. An agent was touring the magazine bureaus of Europe's capitals representing both Blaiberg and his wife. The surgeon who transplanted him was signing contracts for his memoirs and dancing with Gina Lollobrigida in Rome.

On May 2, cardiologist Don Rochelle accompanied Cooley to a medical meeting in Louisiana. Rochelle remembers Cooley speaking disparagingly about transplants. "He said he thought they were being rushed into, that they needed more careful study, that the aura surrounding them was in questionable taste."

Twenty-four hours later, Cooley performed his first heart transplant. Two days after that he did his second. Two days later came his third. Three heart transplants in five days! By the middle of August, he had done ten, more than any surgeon in the world. He was first, undisputably first, and the cameras of *Life* and NBC and the BBC discovered that there was another hospital and another surgeon in Houston to the immediate left of Methodist Hospital and Mike DeBakey.

The nature of heart transplants is that someone has to die in order for someone else to live. But those who succumb to the two leading killers—heart disease and cancer—would not normally have healthy enough hearts left for transfer to someone else. The optimal donor would be a young, previously healthy and vigorous person who died suddenly in an accident that destroyed the brain—but left the heart intact.

At 3 P.M. on Thursday, May 2, 1968, a fifteen-year-old Houston bride, convinced that her nineteen-year-old groom no longer loved her, took a .22 rifle, leaned her head against the barrel, and pulled the trigger. Exploding fragments of lead tore into her brain. She was taken to Ben Taub Hospital's Shock Room, where a team of residents and interns quickly determined that there was no young life left to save. The brain waves were flat, but the heart, strong and vigorous, pumped on, sending blood to an unresponsive and unneeding brain.

Cooley's staff had sent word to Ben Taub that the senior surgeon would appreciate knowing if a potential donor heart turned up, even though the senior surgeon had not yet committed himself with any enthusiasm to a transplant program. Cooley had done but one practice operation, on a cadaver. ("I've done more heart surgery than anyone else in the world," he would say months later to a reporter who inquired how prepared he had been to begin transplants. "I didn't see the value of spending a lot of time in the laboratory putting sutures in dog hearts.") When the news of the girl's suicide reached St. Luke's, two of Cooley's associate surgeons, Grady Hallman and Robert Bloodwell, urged that a transplant take place. The donor heart was across the street and a likely recipient was in the house.

Everett Thomas, a certified public accountant, had come to Houston to see if Denton Cooley could replace three of the four valves in his heart. At 47, Thomas was terrified that another heart attack would take him permanently from his wife and three sons. He had been stricken with scarlet fever during World War II, and had fought the disablement created by his weakened heart for twenty years. He moved to Phoenix for the climate, and took jobs that he could do without strain. Despite his efforts, he had had two heart attacks and two strokes. His heart was failing so severely that the blood supply to his liver was drastically reduced. His liver was swollen and his lungs were not functioning at full capacity and fluids collected in them.

When Cooley returned from the medical meeting in Louisiana, he was told by his associates of Thomas's grave condition. Thomas was scheduled for possible triple-valve replacement on May 3. Cooley was one of the few surgeons in the world who would attempt a triple-valve, but the procedure bore the highest of risks. Cooley also was told that the heart of the bride who had shot herself was available for a possible transplant. The dead and the barely living had come together. Cooley had not sought the situation, but there it was, waiting for his decision. Without committing himself to a transplant, Cooley walked the corridors of the hospital alone. Finally, he made an unexpected call to Thomas's room. Cooley spoke quietly, almost hesitantly. He told Thomas of his extreme heart condition as revealed by the cardiograms and x-rays. He said he would open his heart and examine the valves. "If it seems like I can put in prosthetic valves, then I'll do so. But, on the other hand. . . ."

Cooley's voice trailed off. Thomas and his wife looked at the surgeon anxiously. Cooley began again. Had Thomas and his wife been reading of heart transplants? Both nodded their heads. There was the possibility, Cooley said, of attempting a heart transplant on Thomas, *if* his natural heart would not tolerate replacement valves. There was, he said, a donor heart available. He did not reveal the identity of this heart. Would Thomas and his wife talk over this possibility and let him know within the next few moments? He smiled and left the room hurriedly.

Helen Thomas recalled the moments that followed:

"We had come to Houston with nothing on our mind but a valve operation. We had not even thought of transplants. . . . Dr. Cooley eased us so gently into the idea. We knew that he was not waiting for the opportunity to become a hero, he already was one, so we told him to do what he thought best. He assured us that he would.

"When he left the room, Everett and I talked. Personal things— what a good life we had had, what we were going to do *if.* . . . We weren't optimistic, we weren't fatalistic. We just felt confident that everything would turn out all right . . . whatever that might be. Faith is the big thing. We have to have complete faith in our God. If you allow yourself to worry, then that is not complete faith. Just before Everett went to sleep from the drugs, he took my hand and told me, 'Don't worry about me. If anything happens, you're the one who's going to have troubles. Me, I'm just going to sleep. If I wake up, then everything will be okay.' "

The first heart transplant in Houston was carried out so smoothly that most of the hospital did not even know it was occurring. "It was the quietest one we ever did," recalled Mrs. Ruth Sylvester, supervisor of the operating-room nurses. "All the ones after that we had a hundred medical students and every doctor in the city wanting to watch."

The likelihood that Cooley would transplant a heart caught his staff off guard, most of whom had gone home for the day because it was 6:15 P.M. when Thomas gave his permission. In truth, no one was fully prepared except the surgeon. Mrs. Frances Chandler, an operating-room head nurse, remembers being summoned back to the hospital and driving there at high speed. "I wanted a policeman to stop me so I could tell him I was on my way to do a heart transplant," she said. Mrs. Sylvester, the operating-room supervisor, had been to the beauty parlor and was leaving for a three-day holiday in Mexico when her call came. She hurried to St. Luke's, arriving just after 7 P.M., and immediately began dispatching orders for the scores of tasks that had to be done before the operation could begin.

The most urgent was finding some place to put the patient in—provided he survived the surgery. The Recovery Room was out of the question; totally sterile conditions could not be observed there unless Thomas was the only patient in the room. Cooley did not intend to stop doing other heart surgery just because there was a transplant on his census, nor did the other surgeons who used the crowded facility. There had to be an area close to the surgical suite so that the patient could be rushed back into the operating room quickly, if that became necessary. Mrs. Sylvester came up with the idea of taking one of the operating rooms and converting it into a private recovery room. Cooley agreed. Even as he operated in Room 1, orderlies were taking the standard equipment out of Room 6, cleaning it, sterilizing the walls and floors, bringing in a recovery bed, sterile sheets, monitoring equipment, and every emergency drug Mrs. Sylvester could think of.

Cooley wanted the entire procedure photographed with both still and movie cameras, in both donor and recipient rooms. Mrs. Sylvester called the hospital electrician to make sure there was ample electrical power to accommodate the equipment. The movie photographer would sit on a platform above the operating table and shoot down into Thomas's chest cavity.

Thomas and the girl shared the same blood type, but beyond that there was no time for the more sophisticated tissue typing, which would come with later transplants. Jim Nora had made arrangements to take a sample of blood from both donor and recipient, place them in a specially prepared kit, and fly them to Dr. Paul Terasaki in Los Angeles. There the scientist had facilities to quickly compare the antigens living in white blood cells. Antigens are genetic protein substances that are so tiny as to remain unseen. They aid the body to reject foreign material. Terasaki had discovered at least thirteen antigens (there could be scores more as yet unknown to science) and had devised a method to match up antigens from different blood specimens. He then graded the match from A (blood from identical twins) down to D, the poorest match.

Nora drew blood from Thomas and the girl and dispatched it to Los Angeles, but it was not until the next day—well after the operation was completed—that he learned from Terasaki that the tissue typing was a C match, not good, but, as it would turn out in the months to come, not the worst of those transplants that Cooley would do.

Nor was there time to manufacture ALG, the promising new immunosuppressive drug, which Nora wanted to use in the event that Cooley ever did a transplant. With the operation about to begin, Nora telephoned his friend Dr. Tom Starzl in Denver and asked if he could borrow some, then dispatched his secretary, Nan O'Keefe, in the middle of this frenetic night, to fetch it. Miss O'Keefe, terrified of flight, rode to and from Denver in a thunderstorm, her face white, the precious serum in a styrofoam box clutched between her trembling knees. A plane had crashed the day before and that was the only thing on her mind.

The body of the fifteen-year-old child bride had been transferred from Ben Taub to St. Luke's and placed in Operating Room 2, where a team of doctors and technicians huddled about her. Ironically, Cooley had operated on this same girl to repair an arterial defect when she had been nine years old. Because of their respect and admiration for the surgeon, the girl's parents and her husband gave rapid permission for the transplant. As the ventilator breathed for the technically dead girl, she was given four pints of blood to maintain an adequate pressure. The danger was that the heart would stop if the pressure sank too low, and if the heart stopped it could begin to deteriorate before it was excised and taken across the hall to Room 1, where Thomas would lie.

Shortly before midnight Cooley drank a cup of coffee hurriedly, and with no tension showing, went to the scrub basin. As he cleaned his hands and arms with the disposable soap sponge and his nails with a pointed orange stick, he looked ahead through the glass wall and saw Thomas lying on the table with the anesthesiologist putting him under. Behind Cooley, in Room 2, the girl's heart was rapidly failing. At 12:10 A.M. Grady Hallman called out. The donor heart had stopped and closed chest massage was not bringing it back. Cooley nodded, went hurriedly into Room 1 and opened the heart of Thomas. He saw and felt with his gloved fingers the deterioration of the three valves, calcified and weak. The heart muscle had large sections of scar tissue and a dull gray patch of ischemia, or dead tissue. "There was no doubt that the heart needed replacing," said one who had been present in the room. "But it goes without saying that it would have been considerably anticlimatic to call everything off at that point and just put in three valves."

Word was sent across the hall that Cooley was proceeding with the transplant. Hallman and Bloodwell practically had their scalpels poised. Quickly the girl's chest was opened and the heart exposed, a heart enlarged from the congenital condition, but because of that better suited to fit into a much larger chest. Several months later, in conversation with a visiting scientist from California, Hallman would recall that eerie moment: "You are the one who makes the final blow and takes out the heart and this is a peculiar feeling the first time you do it. . . . I guess just like an executioner who has to pull the switch on the electric chair because it's his job. It bothers him the first time, but the more times he does it, the less it bothers him. . . . It was upsetting to me personally the first time I did it, but the more I did it the easier it became. . . . But the first time you feel as if you are killing the patient. . . ."

Robert Bloodwell removed the entire heart, put it into a stainless steel pan, covered it with a sterile green cloth and carried it the ten feet across the hall to Room 1. Other surgeons believed—and still believe—it is necessary to immediately cool the donor heart and keep it cooled until it is transplanted into the recipient. Cooley had decreed this was not necessary, that a heart could remain in transplantable condition for up to an hour at room temperature.

At 1:01 A.M., Thomas's natural heart was taken from him and put into a container for pathology. The heart-lung bypass machine was working for him. For a few frozen moments, there was the astonishing sight of a man on an operating table, a living man, with nothing but a cavity in the place where his heart should be. Characteristically, Cooley cut the normal operating time for a transplant in half by using a different technique. Others had stitched in a new heart from the outside, having first attached the left atrium of the heart to the base of the left atrium purposely left in place from the patient's old heart. Once this was sewn in place, the technique had been to flop the new heart over to stitch in the right atrium. Other transplanters had left a portion of the back walls of the recipient's atrial chambers, painstakingly cutting out the donor heart to match up with these walls—fitting two jagged puzzle pieces together.

Instead, Cooley reasoned, he could remove the entire heart from the donor, make a bold incision across each atrial chamber to open it up, and suture the new atrial chambers onto the recipient's atrial walls from the *inside*. This technique would also provide enough tissue to make up for any difference between the old heart and the new one. In essence, Cooley would be able to sew faster, and perhaps more important, would not have to flop the new heart about so much as had been necessary before. The less handled, Cooley thought, the less danger there was in damaging it.

By 1:32 A.M., the heart that at dawn the morning before had beat within the chest of a troubled new bride was now sutured into the chest of a weary and frightened accountant from Phoenix. Cooley looked at his work for a few seconds, then said softly that he was going to take Thomas off the bypass pump. Clamps that prohibited blood from flowing into the new heart were removed. Twenty people in the room craned their necks to see what would happen. Frances Chandler, a nurse, held her breath. Another nurse said a silent prayer.

Cooley's hands, holding the defibrillating paddles, were suspended a few inches above the borrowed heart. At least one observer thought his hands were trembling—slightly. Suddenly blood rushed into the arteries of the heart and filled them with the substance of life. Instantly the heart began to fibrillate. Cooley slapped the electric paddles down; one shock stopped the erratic rhythm and sent the heart into a normal, smooth, amazing beat. "Thank God!" someone cried. There was a unanimous whoop inside the operating room. Cooley broke into a wide grin and shook his head as in momentary disbelief. When he had begun his career as a surgeon twenty years before, it was unthinkable to invade the human heart and operate within it. Now he had accomplished the ultimate. It was, he said later, the supreme moment of his life.

By 3 A.M., Thomas's chest was sewn up and he was transferred rapidly to Operating Room 6, transformed into a Recovery Room. At dawn his wife, masked and gowned, was permitted to visit him. Twenty-four hours later, conscious but groggy, he gestured for something to write on. He could not speak with the breathing tube still in his mouth. "What kind of operation did I have?" he wrote in shaky script. His wife told him of his new heart. He wrote hurriedly on the pad again. From whom had the heart come? It was from a young girl who took her life, said Helen Thomas.

"Everett was terribly depressed," she said later that afternoon. "Not about the transplant, but about the child's suicide. He made me tell him all about her, what her troubles were, what caused her to do such a tragic thing."

The news of Cooley's first transplant and the enthusiastic reports on Thomas's postoperative condition spread. Within hours, the phone in Cooley's office started ringing with requests from both referring doctors and patients themselves. Two candidates for heart transplants hurried to Cooley practically on the first plane they could get. One, a 48-year-old school yearbook salesman, James Borden Cobb, of Alexandria, Louisiana, boarded an Air Force plane provided by his congressman. Just before the plane took off, a friend said, "Jim, you may come back from Houston a famous man." Said Cobb, "I don't want to be famous. I just want to live."

The second candidate, James Stuckwish, a 62-year-old hospital administrator from Alpine, Texas, had been a Cooley patient three months earlier but had been rejected for surgery. He had inquired of a transplant but was told that Cooley was not keen on the procedure. As soon as Stuckwish heard of Thomas's new heart, he flew back to Houston. "I've been praying to God that this would happen," he said to Cooley.

Even as the two men settled into the hospital for tests, for waiting, the fates were dealing one of them a heart. A fifteen-year-old boy on a motor scooter collided with a car in Conroe, a town 40 miles north of Houston. Taken to Conroe Hospital, his condition was grave— brain injuries were suspected. The youth was transferred to Methodist Hospital in Houston, where neurologists discovered that the brain was nearly severed from the spinal cord. The EEG was flat. He could not live. Cooley, next door, was promptly notified.

In another of the ironies that marked the transplant era, Cooley had known both the boy and his parents. The mother of the injured teen-ager was active in the "Have-a-Heart" fund in her neighborhood, a social agency that provided wheelchairs, beds, and crutches for the ill and aged. Cooley even had gone to high school with her. He personally asked the woman for her son's heart. She begged to wait, needing counsel from her priest. "I told the family I saw nothing morally against it," said the priest. "I told them I felt it would be the highest act of charity, giving life to another man." The mother, crying, agreed.*

In the years that transplants had been talked of, there had always arisen a hypothetical question: What would the surgeon do if he had one heart and two men in need? Cooley became the first surgeon to face the moral dilemma, only two days after he began his transplant program. Would the 48-year-old school yearbook salesman, or the 62-year-old hospital administrator receive the heart of the fifteen-year-old high school football tackle? Both men had the same blood type as the boy. Once again there was not time enough to fly the blood samples to Los Angeles for a match grade from Terasaki. Cooley wrestled with the decision for most of a day and finally decided that

---

* *Several donor hearts would come from motorcycle victims. Dr. Irvin A. Kraft, a Baylor psychiatrist who made an extensive study of the transplant era, suspected that "donor families . . . viewed their act as one of immolation and sacrifice to shelter themselves from the guilt of having permitted their son to use a motorcycle."*

the younger man would be better able to withstand the procedure.

The operation began at 8:54 P.M. on May 5, and Cooley took only 42 minutes to sew the sturdy adolescent heart * into Cobb's chest. By 11:30 P.M. on the same night, Cobb's blood pressure was satisfactory, his lungs already clearing of fluid, his liver shrinking, his kidneys working well. He was removed to another of the operating rooms that had been transformed into a sterile recovery room. By the time he was able to sit up briefly, he could look into Operating Room 6 and see Everett Thomas giving him a good luck sign and a wave.

Hospital administrator Stuckwish did not have to wait long for his heart. But the one he obtained two days later, on May 7, would be so caught up in a legal and philosophical tangle that the ramifications of the transplant act would not be settled for years, indeed, in some minds and attitudes, never.

---

* *The boy's eyes were donated to the hospital eye bank, and one of his kidneys was transplanted that same night into the body of a 41-year-old man from Odessa, Texas.*

CHAPTER

11

His well-muscled upper right arm was tatooed with a flower and a girl's name, "Fay." On his left, another flower, a bird, a fading heart, and his own name, "Nicks." On the night of April 23, 1968, eleven days before Cooley would do his first transplant, Clarence Nicks was sitting at the bar of the Peek-a-Boo Lounge in the East End section of Houston. He hardly seemed a man of destiny who would soon become the center of a bizarre circus of medical and legal history. Nicks was 32, his nickname "Sonny," and he was a tough, short-tempered welder who drank beer regularly in the cheap and often perilous dives spread along Houston's Ship Channel district. His fellow customers were hard hats, crewmen off the tankers.

On the night that would concern so many, Sonny Nicks was drinking quietly by himself when a friend named McDuffie joined him. McDuffie occasionally worked with Nicks on welding jobs. After a while, McDuffie's estranged wife, later described by the district attorney's office as the "femme fatale" of the evening, came in with two male escorts. McDuffie made a mild attempt at reconciliation, but according to witnesses, was rebuffed. More than an hour passed with the barmaid staying busy opening beer bottles to the accompaniment of blaring country and western music.

Suddenly a brawl erupted over McDuffie's wife, and as many as eight men were fighting beside the bar with Nicks in the thick of the action, the barmaid screaming for them to stop. She ran around the end of the bar and pushed the bunch out the door, slammed it shut, and locked it. Someone inside called the police. Someone outside hit Nicks on the head with a metal object, perhaps a garbage can lid. When the siren of the police car was heard, the brawl stopped. Two investigating officers discovered nothing but Clarence (Sonny) Nicks, who was angry, cursing, and holding a bloody head. Did he know who hit him? Did he want to file charges? "Hell no," Nicks told the officers. "I'll find them bastards next week and charge them myself. . . ."

But because there was an obvious head injury, the officers summoned an ambulance, which took the protesting Nicks to Heights Hospital on the north side of Houston. There he was transferred by his family's request to a smaller suburban hospital where, after a five-day period of observation, he was released on April 28 in the care of his wife and mother. On May 3, the two women had become concerned about Nicks' condition because he "lay around the house sleeping all the time and acting strange." They took him back to the suburban hospital, then across town to Methodist, where neurologists examined his head. At Methodist he fell into a coma, began to deteriorate, and on May 8, a Tuesday, was transferred the hundred yards across to St. Luke's where, shortly before 2 P.M., capping a morning filled with confusion and mystery—his heart was removed and implanted into Henry Stuckwish, the hospital administrator from Alpine.

"I may have to report this operation from prison," Cooley said as he attended to his third transplant in the recovery room. As he spoke, a storm that had been brewing all morning across the Medical Center in the basement of Ben Taub Hospital broke with fury.

The medical examiner of Harris County is Dr. Joseph Jachimczyk, whose territory is one of the largest—476 square miles—and most violent in America. Until he became examiner—or coroner—in 1956, the Houston metropolitan area had no such officer. It was the principal American city that had no modern coroner system. Violent and mysterious deaths were investigated by a justice of the peace, who was not required by law to be a man possessed of medical knowledge. When a drowning or a shooting or a traffic death was reported by police, the justice of the peace would go to the scene, be shown a body, and declare that the man was certainly dead. Often the justice of the peace was accompanied by a surgical or pathology resident from Baylor who could advise him in making a decision as to death. The residents were eager to assist for two reasons: (1) to practice autopsy and (2) to obtain sections of the aorta, which both DeBakey and Cooley were using in such huge numbers during the early and mid-1950s, sewing them into living patients before the plastic ones became available. This was one reason why DeBakey was able to report such astonishingly large series of successful aneurysm operations in that period. He could depend upon a continuing supply of re-usable aortas from the violent deaths of his city. There was nothing illegal in the practice. Moreover, no one ever knew about the custom except the resident who did the autopsy, snipped out the material, and sewed up the chest before burial. Some of the aortas were used instantly, others kept in an antibiotic solution, chilled and kept up to ten days, still others freeze-dried and kept indefinitely.

The first thing Jachimczyk did when he took office in 1956 was to institute a modern and scientific examination procedure to rule on the cause of death. "There is no question in my mind that many many homicides were passed off by my predecessors as 'coronary thrombosis,'" he once said, "when in fact the 'thrombosis' was caused by an ice-pick hole in the chest." In the decade and a half that followed, Jachimczyk was frequently in the headlines, quarreling with local governments over funds he demanded to enlarge and staff his facilities, or sitting in a courtroom witness box and devouring a defense attorney who dared to challenge his findings. Quite simply, he was not a man to tamper with; Jachimczyk held both medical *and* legal degrees. He also courted the press of Houston, relishing, as did so many others in the city, his name in type. Since he had come to the city, he felt he had seen—and investigated—every kind of death that the mind of man could conceive and commit. But "The Case of the Heartless Corpse," as he was to call it in a scientific paper concerning Clarence Nicks, was beyond even *his* imagination.

All during that first week of May, 1968, Jachimczyk had been annoyed at Cooley and his staff. "His first donor heart was from a girl who committed suicide," he recalled later. "That girl had been brought into Ben Taub Hospital with a gunshot wound in her head. Somehow Dr. Bloodwell on Cooley's staff heard about her being there—and she was whisked out of here before I or anybody knew it. And my office is in the basement of Ben Taub! Why was this girl taken out of this hospital in the middle of the night? What did they have to hide? No one even asked me if she could be removed.

"Dr. Milam, the pathologist at St. Luke's, did have the courtesy to telephone me and mention that there was a possibility she might become a donor. But I learned later that the transplant was already in progress, even as we talked on the telephone."

Jachimczyk began to feel that the surgeons were running end sweeps on him. "I'd always tried to cooperate with those guys," he complained. "They call over and say, for example, 'I need a piece of femur for a patient who is approximately six feet, two inches, tall, etc., etc., etc.,' and if a body came in over the weekend that matched up, we'd cut out a piece of bone in autopsy and send it over. We did the same thing with corneas and cartilage. We always looked in a fellow's wallet to see if he had one of those donor cards that said he wanted to give his body or any part of it to science."

When the medical examiner arrived at work on the morning of May 8, 1968, he received an immediate telephone call from a homicide officer at police headquarters in downtown Houston. Did Jachimczyk know anything of one Clarence (Sonny) Nicks, believed to be the victim of a barroom brawl? Was he dead or alive? Jachimczyk had never heard of the man and routinely began dialing the hospitals of the Medical Center. He discovered quickly that Nicks was that very morning a patient at St. Luke's, having been recently transferred from two previous hospitals. "They told me at St. Luke's that Nicks was alive," said Jachimczyk, "and I lost interest. My jurisdiction begins at the time of death."

At mid-morning, Dr. Lind, a pathologist at St. Luke's, telephoned the medical examiner and said Nicks was being considered as a potential heart donor. Jachimczyk's back shot up. "I cautioned Dr. Lind against it," he said later. "In fact, I *warned* him against it. I did not feel a homicide case should be used in the transplant program. Cooley and his boys had been planning to do these transplants since

January and they had totally overlooked the medical examiner's office. My office would have to be their major source of donated organs!"

At 11:05 A.M.—Jachimczyk keeps meticulous records of phone calls—he was notified by Dr. Pedro Carem, the physician who had been Nicks' private doctor and who had accompanied him on an odyssey through four Houston hospitals, that the welder was indeed dead. "At *that* point," Jachimczyk remembered, "it became my case."

But no sooner had he put down the phone than it rang again, this time the caller being Bloodwell of the Cooley team. *He* assured Jachimczyk that Nicks was *not* dead, but was still a potential heart donor.

"I had no choice," said Jachimczyk, "I had to believe Bloodwell. I couldn't look askance at the word of a duly licensed physician or osteopath. But I was damn confused by this time. The press had gotten word of Cooley's plan to use a homicide victim's heart—if indeed there was a homicide victim—and they were clamoring to know what I was going to do. I decided the best thing I could do would be to get some ground rules laid down."

Out went urgent messages to the district attorney's office, prominent physicians, lawyers, hospital administrators, and city and county officials. A meeting was to be held under emergency conditions for 1 P.M. that day. In between the flood of calls, Cooley himself telephoned Jachimczyk—an hour before the scheduled conference. Sonny Nicks was still alive, said Cooley, but his brain waves were flat. For all intents and purposes, the surgeon said, the man was dead.

"Nonetheless, I strongly urge you not to use this man's heart," snapped Jachimczyk, his temper barely in check. "This is a homicide situation. Do you understand that?"

"This is also a desperate situation," answered Cooley in an emotional appeal. "I have a recipient (Stuckwish) waiting, and prepared. We cannot turn down this man's chance at getting a heart."

Exasperated, Jachimczyk repeated what he had been saying so strongly all morning. He reminded Cooley that a meeting in less than an hour would lay down ground rules to avoid future dilemmas.

"Well," Cooley said, "I'm glad you're having the meeting, but I feel I'll probably have to go ahead with what we have planned."

Jachimczyk paused. He did not want to get in the way of medical progress. He merely wanted his rules followed. "If it will help any," he said, "I won't press charges against you. But I cannot guarantee that nobody else will."

The meeting began at 1 P.M. While the committee discussed the legal issues of transplantation, Bloodwell was removing Sonny Nicks' heart and carrying it across the hall in a steel pan where Cooley implanted it into Stuckwish. "I foolishly wondered at the time why Denton did not attend our meeting," said Jachimczyk.

Throughout the year that followed, the medical examiner tilted with Cooley. Jachimczyk made formal pleas to both Cooley and to DeBakey—who had not yet begun transplantation—urging them not to use homicide hearts. DeBakey quickly agreed; Cooley declined, saying he would use any and all donor hearts if an emergency situation presented itself. His primary consideration, he said, was for the living, not the dead.

"I think I must hold the world record for heartless corpses at autopsy," Jachimczyk said ruefully as the year neared its end. "After the third one, it really began to upset me. And I wasn't the only man in my field with the problem. My counterpart in Los Angeles telephoned me long distance and complained that Cooley had flown a body to Houston and was using its heart. I told him, 'That's not my bother, you shouldn't have let your corpse get out of town.' "

The district attorney's office spent more than six months investigating the death of Clarence Nicks and in January, 1969, obtained a grand jury indictment against two young laborers who were charged with murder. The indictment charged that Robert Damon Patterson and Alfred Lee Branum ". . . with malice aforethought did kill Clarence Nicks by beating and striking him with fists and a can and by kicking with their feet and by such other means, instruments, or weapons unknown to the grand jury." No action was brought against Cooley or any member of his staff.

Almost two years later, in the autumn of 1970, the case had not yet come to trial. Attorney Hal Hudson, representing Patterson, was eager for trial. He was a young, ambitious lawyer who had caught lightning in a bottle. "My client, Mr. Patterson, is a good kid," he told a visitor in the summer of 1970. "He has no previous felony convictions or misdemeanors involving moral turpitude. I will claim in my defense that Clarence Nicks, not my client, instigated the argument which led to the fight at the Peek-a-Boo Lounge."

The lawyer had a stack of medical books and scientific papers on his desk. He had been reading up on heart transplants. He had, in case the self-defense theory failed, a sensational backstop.

"I will also ask the question, 'What is death?' " he said, "and, perhaps more relevant, '*When* is death?' Clarence Nicks was pronounced dead twice, perhaps three times the morning of May 8, 1968.

"I wonder if Clarence Nicks might still be alive today if his heart had not been cut from his chest. I have seen movies of a heart-transplant operation. The way the surgeons tell it, the donor heart is barely palpitating. But the way I saw it, and the way a jury will see it, the heart is beating like a bass drum! *Whomp! Whomp! WHOMP!* You gonna tell me that sum bitch is dead when his heart is a-whompin' away like that? You show that whompin' heart to a jury and you think for one minute they'll consider this to be a murder victim?"

Attorney Hudson paused and smiled. Then he frowned. He leaned forward and addressed an imaginary jury:

"I don't think we've gotten to the point where doctors can declare somebody a vegetable and then drop the executioner's ax on him!"

CHAPTER
12

Two of Cooley's first three transplants died quickly—yearbook salesman Cobb of infection within three days; hospital administrator Stuckwish from a variety of complications ranging from blood clots to liver malfunction within six days. The controversial heart of Sonny Nicks had functioned normally, but in vain.

Cooley's first transplant, the remarkable Everett Thomas, overcame a brief period of rejection, a touch of jaundice, and moved almost hurriedly to what seemed would be total recovery and acceptance by his system of the new heart. There was one early distasteful moment when the nineteen-year-old widower of the girl whose heart had been donated decided that he should receive money for his generosity. "He sort of demanded that Thomas pay him regular rent on the heart!" exclaimed one of the nurses. The news was leaked to the newspapers and radio, and despite the nurses' attempts to keep the ghoulish report from Everett Thomas, he announced one morning that he knew a price had been put on his new heart. "It doesn't bother me," he assured the nurses. "I have no attachment to this heart at all. It's just a pump, after all. I came to St. Luke's Hospital just like it was a store and they could have had this heart on a shelf for all I care. I bought it like any other piece of merchandise."

The fourth day after his operation, Thomas was walking and taking solid food. He said he felt like a man getting over nothing more serious than the flu. "I'm a little weak in the legs," he said, "but I haven't felt this good in years." Suddenly he broke into tears. "Dr. Cooley has been named Man of the Year by a lot of organizations. . . . All I can say is that he is . . . he is . . . he's the man of my life."

Everyone noticed that a change had come over Denton Cooley. He never had been comfortable in the spotlight, but suddenly he was giving interviews, appearing on television, posing with Christiaan Barnard at transplant seminars and seemingly enjoying every moment of it. He remarked in conversation to a visiting psychiatrist from Los Angeles, "The most stimulating experience in my professional life was the completion of our first transplant . . . to see that organ begin to function again in a new body. As a consequence, unfortunately I guess, but in some ways fortunately, I as a personality was vaulted into some sort of orbit where they thought I was some kind of super-surgeon. . . . It was fantastic! The reaction that the public and the news media had was fantastic. We were dealing with the heart! We were taking one man's heart and putting it into another. Every day we put in three or four mechanical valves into peoples' hearts and nobody got excited about it, but do a heart transplant, and overnight the surgeon becomes some sort of diety!"

Don Rochelle, the boyish-looking cardiologist who was asked by Cooley to serve with Jim Nora as immunologist for the transplants, remembered the first three months of the transplant year—May, June, July—as being a time of "tremendous euphoria."

"Denton was willing to transplant everybody," said Rochelle. "Of our first nine, three were almost dead when they went into surgery, they never really stood a chance. Denton took 'em on anyway—to hell with the statistics! To the surgeon, it was almost akin to really being God. It was a feeling of rare *ecstasy* that enveloped Denton. He was given the power to grant life!" That the surgeon had jumped completely ahead of the rest of medicine was something that would not become obvious for a few months to come.

Two rooms at the end of Three South in St. Luke's were converted into a special transplant suite. The hospital carpenters built an anteroom, which shut off the suite from the rest of the floor. Cooley wanted a special nurse to run the transplant suite and supervise the care of his star patients, a strawboss of super efficiency who would not fear these extraordinary people. The transplants were becoming such celebrated residents of the hospital that some nurses were frankly loath to work with them, fearing a nursing error might bring down the wrath of all the doctors involved. One of the supervisors thought of Alice Nye.

Alice was a splendid choice. Steel-backed, with a rich booming contralto, she was the kind of nurse anyone really sick would want to have—feminine enough to mother you, tough enough to know when to sympathize and when to bark. During World War II, she was a first lieutenant who had won a battlefield decoration for bravery in the Normandy campaign. She had come to Houston in the late 1940s and vividly remembers being scrub nurse for one of Mike De-Bakey's very first operations. DeBakey had come up with a new theory that if lap packs were hot enough, they would cauterize blood vessels. He wanted them dipped in boiling hot saline solution just before they were handed to him. Alice stood next to the surgeon, expected to pass him his surgical instruments and at the same time dip the lap packs into pans of steaming water borne in by a procession of orderlies. Her hands turned lobster red inside her gloves, followed by her temper, and she finally announced, in battlefield terminology, that she could not do both efficiently. Even Mike DeBakey accepted what Alice said.

Alice had trained at a sprawling hospital in Shreveport, Louisiana, and had set high personal standards for herself. But modern medicine had changed in the three decades since she had learned her art. "When I started out as a nurse, I was perfectly capable of handling 26 patients on a floor at one time," she said, "but medicine grew so fast that I found I just couldn't do it my way any more. I didn't want some nurse's aid to take the blood pressure of a critically ill patient because I was busy with something else, or some licensed vocational nurse to give medicine and write up charts. Rather than do less than what I forced myself to do, I quit hospital work and went into private-duty nursing."

But she was intrigued by the offer to boss the transplant suite. Quickly she confessed that she knew little of how to handle them. "Who does?" was the answer.

In the year that followed, Alice would become more than a nurse: she was mistress of the moon landing and sometimes head of a nursery. She became emotionally involved with her brood—arbiter of heated jealousies among the transplanted hearts—and in some cases their families. She spent the last few desperate months tending to dying people and telling lies as well and as fast as she could. Her philosophy always had been: "I want everybody to get well, I want to win them all." But she lost them all, and not until the last was gone did she have the time to break. And cry.

On the first day Alice discovered that transplants were terrified if there was the slightest deviation in care and routine. Her initial hours on the job were spent in listening to Everett Thomas announce and lecture to her how things should be done for him, how the other nurses had taken his temperature and read his monitoring devices, and when he had received his shots and pills. Alice assured him that she had the ability to nurse him well. Patients began squealing on doctors who walked into their rooms without wearing sterile gowns, caps, and masks. There was a running battle with Leachman over his cigar that Alice never did win. "Dr. So and So just came in without a mask," one would complain to Alice. "That's all right," she would answer wryly, "They're all sterile doctors around here, anyway."

It was a year of doctor pitted against doctor, nurse against nurse, a year of resurrection, a year of grotesque horror. At one point in deepest autumn, more than twenty people were camped in motels scattered about Cooley's hospital, all waiting for new hearts, all waiting for Cooley's hands to open their chests and install them there, waiting on fretful motel beds, eyes to the telephone, ears to the open windows—better to hear the ambulance when it sped out South Main to the Medical Center. The cry of an ambulance meant that somewhere in the city someone had been shot or run over or crushed in a fall, and if that someone was dead or dying, perhaps the heart would still be usable. When the ambulance broke the quiet autumn nights, the waiters—as they were called—sat up in their motel beds and switched on bedside lights and stared hard at the telephone . . . and waited to be summoned across the street to the hospital for tests. "For a hundred nights I prayed," said the wife of a man now long dead, "let tonight be the night that Sonny will get his new heart."

By July 30, 1968, Cooley had transplanted nine hearts, and six of the owners—five men and one woman—appeared beside him triumphant. They posed for photographs with Cooley, who stood proud as a schoolmaster. Cooley's sudden penchant for publicity surprised many Houston doctors. One, a veteran cardiologist, analyzed it carefully. "The odd thing," he told a visitor months after the hysteria had passed, "is that in the early years, Cooley was a white hat, a supporter of the medical society and its ethics regarding publicity. He disapproved of DeBakey's pursuit of print. I feel Denton sat down with himself one night and decided that the only way to get funds for his Texas Heart Institute was through publicity—and to ride it out through hell and high water. I think he made this decision carefully, consciously. To become a star in medicine, you needed a gimmick. And he had been taught by a master."

Everett Thomas was well enough to leave the hospital, but not the city, so he found work in the trust department of a bank directly across from St. Luke's. Louie Fierro, Cooley's fourth transplant, found the same work he had done in Yonkers, New York—selling used cars. After his operation Cooley had said to him, "You are the only used-car salesman in the world who ever had a change of heart." Garrulous and friendly, Fierro had become a great favorite of the hospital staff. He spoke in the rapid style of Eastern America and he usually had a blue joke for any nurse he met.

Though released from the hospital, Thomas and Fierro were bound to it—medically and emotionally. They were instructed to return officially at least three days a week for shots, EKGs, x-rays, and blood tests by Nora or Rochelle. But almost every morning they began their day by looking in on Alice and the exclusive sterile club she ran. They came to make "rounds." They put on cap, gown, masks, and paper boots over their shoes and they questioned Alice in the manner of doctors. "How's the new guy doing?" they would demand. "How's his pulse? How's his respiration? Is he taking his Kickapoo Joy Juice?"—Alice's term for the daily solu-curtef (a cortisone derivative) injections.

Those with new hearts became the new celebrities. Lives of pain and dullness and fear, of being confined to a back bedroom with drawn shades and a night stand crowded with bottles and solutions, were transformed by Cooley's knife into lives of dazzle and acclaim. Each kept scrapbooks and autograph albums beside his bed. Their mail was enormous; one had stamps from 37 countries. Kings and leaders of government visited them, congratulated them, offered prayers for them.

Don Rochelle noted that they became "evangelists, almost as the Twelve Apostles went out to tell of the wondrous thing that had happened to them." Everett Thomas had been a quiet, retiring, shy man, but with his new heart he was transformed into a social lion, comfortable on the dais, accustomed to the microphone, familiar to the Rotarians and Kiwanians of South Texas. Television cameras captured Louie Fierro patting fenders at his used car lot. Carl Van Bates, shoe salesman from Amarillo, became so passionate over his new heart that he wrote fellow golfer Dwight David Eisenhower a letter as the stricken President lay in Walter Reed Hospital in Washington, D.C. Ike should come to Houston, Van Bates wrote, and let the hands of Denton Cooley give him a new heart, a new life. Alice obtained a putter and a golf ball and rigged up a styrofoam cup for Van Bates to practice putting in his hospital room. They became exhibits A, B, C, D, E, and F for the most astonishing operation—in the public eye —since medicine began.

Philip Blaiberg was one faraway hero. Every time he was photographed riding a bicycle on a Cape Town lane or plunging into the surf, that clipping became, to the Houston transplants, almost as sacred as a religious icon. Denton Cooley was the other. Even though the surgeon had little to do with managing the transplants in the critical postoperative weeks, each owner of a new heart identified strongly with him. Though fifteen physicians—from dermatologist to inhalation specialist to radiologist—were often intimately involved with the care of a transplant, Dr. Kraft, the Baylor psychiatrist said, "The patients always conceptualized themselves as being the surgeon's patients. Thus, at each step of the stairway to transplantation and the subsequent war with rejection, the patients felt constantly the highly charged impact of the personality and charisma of the surgeon."

Merely by walking into their room for a few moments, Cooley

elated his people. He was the producer of the film dropping into the dressing room of the starring actor, and, indeed, each case had been filmed before, during, and after his transplant. Each cherished Cooley's public comments as insurance for his transformation.

"There is no question in my mind that heart transplants can be done with very low risk—say 5 percent mortality," he said during the period of euphoria. "It will become a routine operation during the next decade. The clinical feasibility has already been established. It's only a question now of resolving such details as body rejection and getting people to accept the idea of walking around with someone else's heart."

On another occasion Cooley remarked, "People might wonder what life with another person's heart would be like after the initial risk of the operation is past. After all, the heart has long been considered the seat of the soul and the objects of poets and songs. I believe the best way to think of life is that every organ in the body is a servant to the brain. Once the brain is gone the servant is unemployable. Then we must find these organs other employment."

When he was criticized at one medical meeting for transplanting hospital administrator Stuckwish, who had suffered one cardiac arrest in the hours before his surgery and a second attack even as the doctors cut into his chest on the table, Cooley answered sharply, "There are few surgeons in the world who would try what we did on Stuckwish. We don't refuse to operate on patients if they are too sick, only if they're not sick enough. The real issue here is not are we going to offer a transplant to a man, but are we going to deny it to someone who is in the last hour of his life!" The fact that Stuckwish died within a few days of the transplant was less relevant, Cooley said, than the fact that the transplant resuscitated him and gave him those few more days of life. "Stuckwish's case illustrates dramatically that a transplant has real therapeutic clinical value," he said. "We have demonstrated that resuscitation of a patient by transplant is possible."

There were even words from the surgeon to gladden those camped out in the motels waiting for hearts. Rumbling was heard in the medical world that transplants were becoming a carnival of false hope. Many doctors were pleading for a moratorium to examine and contemplate what was happening. "Nonsense," said Cooley. "We don't have enough patients done yet to assess the results. Every case that is attempted proves the validity of the concept."

But the new moon turned and by autumn its dark side came into view.

Within every human body dwells a defense mechanism to protect the body against foreign intrusion. Let the thumb pick up a splinter and instantly the mechanism goes into action, examining the sliver of wood, deciding it is not "self" but "non-self" and taking steps to expel it.

When the surgeon puts a foreign heart into a body, the defense mechanism is outraged. The transplanted heart leaks antigens, those indicators of genetic difference, into the new system. They begin to explore the strange new environment. Antigens hurry to the lymph nodes, which in turn promptly manufacture antibodies and immune competent lymphocytes to wage war against these unknown invaders. The body is sending out "self" to repel "non-self." The antibodies and immune competent lymphocytes rush to the new heart—the source of these antigens—and chew it up, immobilize it, reject it.

The defense mechanism not only works against transplanted hearts; it is there to guard against infection, viruses, any foreign threat to the body. After the surgeon had done his quick work, the cardiologists faced the maddening problem of how to slow down and stall off the rejection process against the new heart, but at the same time not cripple the mechanism so drastically that the body had no strength to battle pneumonia or infection. It loomed eminently possible that a transplant patient could be treated with enough drugs to permit his system to accept the new heart, but he might die of a common cold.

To Jim Nora and Don Rochelle, with help from the entire St. Luke's cardiology staff, Leachman, Dennis Cokkinos, and Louis Leatherman among others, fell the complex task of managing rejection. There was no principle that cut across the body of their work, because each system was different, each patient reacted differently to the drugs. "After a while, it got to the point where we would say, 'Well, let's try this or that and see what happens,'" said one of the heart doctors. "Every day was a new ball game."

The names of the cardiologists were rarely if ever in newspapers, but their lives were far more deeply entwined with the bearers of the new hearts than the surgeon himself. Rochelle estimated he saw the transplants up to twenty-five times every day.

Nora and Dr. John Trenton of Baylor had quickly begun a program of making ALG, the immunosuppressive drug that seemed the most promising in control of rejection. Its preparation was interesting. During open-heart surgery, Cooley would remove a piece of the thymus from some patient, usually a child, and send it to Nora. The thymus, which begins to atrophy when a person becomes fourteen and eventually disappears, is a key organ for cellular immunity. The thymus was then ground down into a serum that was injected into a horse. "Usually," said Nora, "a mangy, old, broken-down nag we bought for $10 and boarded at a stable across town." The first such horse used, a sway-back called Preacher, received injections of the thymus serum over a period of several days. At the end of six weeks, during which time Preacher's system had been manufacturing antibodies, two quarts of blood were drained from an artery in his leg and processed in the Baylor laboratories. Through sophisticated distillation, the horse blood was reduced to ALG—a drug whose most valuable components were the horse antibodies—and administered to the human transplant patients. The need for ALG became so immense, because of the large number of Cooley's patients, that the process had to be speeded up and the horses sacrificed rather than drained. From thirty quarts of blood in a full-grown horse, five quarts of ALG were obtained.

The transplants also received massive shots of steroids—chemical relatives of those hormones made by the human adrenal gland. Steroids such as cortisone have a general immunosuppressive reaction, but they can have bizarre side effects.

With the first large doses of cortisone, the typical transplant patient became positively euphoric. "Many said they suddenly had no pain at all, not even in the thoracic incision," said Rochelle. "After this God-awful operation, to have no pain!"

But a week later, many became depressed, and for brief periods psychotic. Some had total withdrawal, lying mute, catatonic in their beds, staring out at a blank unknown that only they could see. Others burst into tears for no apparent reason. One sobbed so hysterically that his wife and child began to cry as well, and tranquilizers had to be administered to all. Some were unable to eat. Others had memory lapses. Alice handed one patient his toothbrush and he looked at it with such total bewilderment that she had to demonstrate what he was supposed to do with it. Some could not move their limbs. Some could not sleep, others *would* not sleep. To close the eyes was to die, in the mind of one transplant. Nora grew weary of having his telephone ring in the middle of the night and hearing the familiar story from the charge nurse, of dressing and driving to the hospital, of coaxing the man with the new heart to sleep, sitting beside his bed, holding his hand, assuring him that another morning would surely come.

One patient sat in a chair near the window with his rosary and rocked from side to side. Alice hesitated to interrupt his prayers until she observed that he was staring blankly at the wall. He was in a stupor. The same man was careful not to turn on his left side. He was afraid that the new heart would fall from its place.

During one rejection episode, a patient was given greater dosages of prednisone, a cortisone derivative, and the resulting euphoria built in his mind a kind of spirit. He called it "lamade" and for a few days it dominated his life. A Baylor psychiatrist interviewed him:

Examiner: "What is this lamade?"

Patient: "A beautiful thing. Off and on. This is ozone. That's as far as I can go. Off and on. Off and on. Beautiful." (He began to laugh loudly.)

Examiner: "I notice there's a scar on your chest." (Pointing to the incision for the transplanted heart)

Patient: "I had a cancer."

Examiner: "Is there anything under the skin?"

Patient: "No. All empty."

Examiner: "If I put this stethoscope on and listen there, what will I hear?"

Patient: "Lamade . . . that's all."

Examiner: "Where's your heart?"

Patient: "You are my heart." (He burst into tears.)

Before his transplant, one patient of German ancestry had been a gentle barber. After he received his new heart, for brief periods of time, he turned into a loud and troublesome anti-Semite. He raged at the "rich kike friends" of a fellow transplant, he cursed Jews with such venom that Alice finally scolded him. It almost seemed that the surgeon had nicked a hidden sac and out spilled a lifetime of latent hatred.

At three one morning, a transplant filled his bathtub with water and prepared to enter it, whistling, singing, oblivious to the blackness outside his window and the silence of the hospital. Across the hall of the transplant suite, a patient heard the noise and rang for the night nurse. She ordered the bather back to bed. From that moment on, the two patients were bitter enemies. Later, when the informer died, the bather heard the news and sprang from his bed, rushing down the hall and telling each patient to leave the hospital. "We will all die," he cried. "Flee!" Alice took the bather by the hand, marched him to his room, calmed him, and sternly commanded him to go to each room and apologize.

Disorientation, confusion, and memory lapses seldom lasted more than a few days, although all could return with altered dosages of cortisone. But there was another side effect that no one liked. Their faces swelled up like balloons. "If I were in a crowd of 20,000 people at Madison Square Garden, I could spot a transplant," said one doctor. "Their faces began to haunt me."

Several of the transplanted men felt awakened virility. One casually left his pajama bottoms open and exposed himself as Alice entered and left his room. She ignored it at first but finally became annoyed and asked him to fasten his pants. "Oh, I'm just a participant in the hospital transplant program, and you're a member of the hospital staff," the man said with an injured look. "It shouldn't bother you." "Well it does," said Alice. "And to tell the truth, it isn't all that interesting." Another patient who had been impotent for many years because of his failing heart almost proudly demonstrated an erection after his transplant.

"Virility and courage," said Dr. Kraft, the psychiatrist, "seem to be traits the patients associate with the new heart."

Some male patients, said Kraft, expressed concern about receiving hearts from female donors. One patient told his daughter, "Now I am a woman." Another referred to his new heart, in conversations with Kraft, as his "lady," answering questions about himself in the female gender.

As the barber with anti-Semitic outbursts prepared to return to his home in a Southern state, he approached Alice in the corridor and, in the manner of the violin teacher in a famous perfume ad, bent her backward and kissed her on the mouth. "I've always wanted to do that," he said. Alice was an unwilling student. She wrenched free and hit him hard in the chest with an Army-nurse punch. "Oh God," she thought as she did it, "I hope I don't knock his transplanted heart loose." Months later she received a long-distance telephone call that the barber was rejecting and she hung up the telephone in despair. "Nobody in his town knows how to nurse a transplant," she said. "Everybody is sick, the whole world is caving in on my patients."

Alice Nye knew she was violating a cardinal rule of nursing, but her life became deeply entwined with the patients and their families. Not content with working shifts that sometimes stretched to twelve and fourteen hours, seven days a week, she spent her time away from the hospital running errands for her transplants, finding apartments for their families, buying groceries and altering the bill so that she would receive but one-half reimbursement. Her shoulder was large enough for the wives to weep when they no longer could accept or understand what their husbands were going through. She told bawdy jokes, she played honky-tonk piano, she invited the celebrated new hearts to her home and stuffed them with boiled crabs and steak and beer. Alice was mother to them all. She was social worker, therapist, fun and games director, and—always—intense watcher; even when her eyes were merry and her face was wreathed in the boisterousness of a joke or a song, she was watching.

The first storm clouds appeared in early November, 1968. Everett Thomas, six months into his new and celebrated life, walked into St. Luke's and told Don Rochelle, "I feel punk." He could not button his trousers because his abdomen was sore. He did not know that his liver was enlarged, that his new heart was not supplying it with enough blood because it was battling to keep from being rejected. Both Rochelle and Nora were immediately worried, but they attempted to mask their alarm. "Everett Thomas was a man we had watched almost every day," said Rochelle, "and when he came in and said, 'I feel punk,' it frightened us."

Two nights later car salesman Fierro was dining at the home of Alice Nye and her husband. Fierro had become a frequent and welcome guest. Alice's husband, a grocery manager, remembers Fierro as "a man's man, a fellow who enjoyed a good joke, a good drink, a bet now and then; he was a man who found his new life full and beautiful." He was also a man who denied the symptoms of rejection that were assaulting his heart. On this night another guest in the Nye home was a former wrestler named Vigali, who owned the nearby Big Humphrey Pizza Parlor. Vigali and fellow Italian Fierro had become close friends.

At dinner, Alice began to worry. Her patient was scratching his wrists and hands over and over again, something he had not done before. His eyes were puffed and sunken. It obviously pained him to walk across the room, but he denied any discomfort. He even snapped at his good friend, Vigali, for suggesting that he felt less than par.

"Louie," ordered Alice, trying to keep her voice good-natured, "you're so damned grouchy tonight, lemme listen to your new heart." Alice kept a stethoscope and blood-pressure cuff in her home. She felt her own heart leap as she listened to Fierro's. It sounded labored; his pulse had a sharp, crackling tone, its rate approached 150. The blood pressure was dangerously low.

"I tried to hide my horror," remembered Alice. "I tried to get him to go to the hospital that very night. I made up every lie I could think of without alarming him. He said he was due to go in the next morning, anyway, first thing. I insisted that he get there early and be first so that the doctors would have more time and he wouldn't have to wait."

Alice slept little that night. The next day, Fierro did not appear at the hospital until after lunch. He had vomited the entire morning, yet he had stayed home to watch himself on television selling cars. Because Thomas had been put in the sterile unit, and because there was another transplant being nursed in the second room, Fierro had to be put down the hall in regular floor care.

Nora and Rochelle fought Fierro's rejection for 48 hours without sleep. Alice had no nursing responsibility toward Fierro because he was not in her special unit anymore, but when her shift was over, she hovered outside his door. "I heard him calling for me," she said. "I went into his room and he was begging for ice. They're always thirsty toward the end. . . . Nobody was there at the moment and I opened his oxygen tent and reached into his ice bucket and I got a good handful of that soft, mushy ice, and I opened his mouth and stuffed it in and watched him work it down. I closed the tent and left the room. It was the last favor I ever did for Louie. I ran out of the hospital and by the time I was home, the phone was ringing, and Louie was dead."

For a month, the fight to save Thomas was waged. Instantly an intravenous drip was started, rushing to his system big doses of steroids and Immural. His blood pressure fell to 75 over 60, perilously narrow. His symptoms of rejection would become familiar. Only in rejection did the transplants follow a pattern:

1. A rubbing sound over the heart caused by friction and fluid within the pericardial sac. This sometimes happens in open-heart surgery, but it usually goes away. With transplants, it did not.

2. EKG changes: loss of voltage, changes in the T waves.

3. Elevation in one enzyme of the heart muscle, the LDH 1 enzyme, indicating that the heart muscle was damaged and leaking the enzyme into the blood stream.

4. Breathing difficulty.

5. Liver enlargement.

6. Malaise. As Thomas had said, "I feel punk."

When everything seemed to fail, when the immunologists could not beat back the rejection eating away at Thomas's new heart, Cooley suddenly announced a bold decision. He would transplant Thomas *again*. He would give him another new heart. He presented the idea to the gravely ill accountant. His reaction? "Resignation," remembered Nora. "He said, in effect, 'I've gone this far with you fellows.' "

Thomas became the first man in history to have had three hearts within his chest—the one he was born with, the one he borrowed from a child suicide and lived with for six months, and the one he died with. He rejected on Cooley's table during his second heart transplant, and on the third postoperative day, died. Nora assumed he was sensitized to some antigens in the second transplanted heart that had not been discovered.

A wave of uneasiness swept the world of the new hearts. Some of those waiting in the motel rooms packed and went away. Cooley had done eighteen transplants by November 30, 1968, but ten were dead and others were failing. The warmth of the summer had a cold breeze blowing against it. "There was supportive interaction among the transplants and the waiters," said Nora. "But mainly it was the kind of relationship like one might have seen in the Warsaw ghetto during World War II." Who would be next? was the question. And when he died, "Ah, but *he* was a bad match," or "But *he* didn't cooperate with the doctors," or "But *he* had no will to live." Nothing, however, was uttered with high enthusiasm. In addition to the scrapbooks of Blaiberg laughing and the headlines of joyful new life, the Houston transplants began keeping scorecards—who was transplanted, how long he lived, when he died, of what he died. Early in the program there had been jealousy among the transplants as to who could stay in Alice's transplant suite with the wall-to-wall carpeting and plush furnishings. When a patient was moved down the hall to regular nursing care, often he complained of second-class status. Psychiatrist Kraft noted that when the rejection and death become common, "the transplant suite changed its symbolism from the womb-like core center getting its occupants prepared for a new birth of freedom to the place where you went when assaulted by rejection, perhaps not to emerge alive again."

One patient demanded that doctors and visitors put on *three* masks when they entered his room, so terrified was he of germs. Another transplant shared a room with a man whose heart was rejecting. When doctors and nurses surrounded his bed and began to work with only a beige curtain drawn about them, the first transplant paid little heed. Then he turned on his radio and attached an ear plug and heard with mounting alarm a news announcer broadcast that the man in the next bed was dying of rejection. Another patient heard of his *own* rejection from a television newscast.

One transplant suffered the horror of having his face chewed away by herpes virus. His body resistance was so lowered by the immuno-suppressive drugs that the disease ran rampant. Whenever he fell fitfully asleep, Alice would creep silently into his room and bathe the black scabs with peroxide and try to remove them. The patient had been a splendid-looking man but could no longer even bear to look at himself in the mirror. She worked the longest on his nose. By the time he died, Alice had done her work: there were no more black scabs, not even on his nose. In his last hours, as he lay in terminal failure, Alice urged him to keep trying, to fight for more life. "I'll try one more day," he gasped, "but then I'll give up." Fifteen minutes later he was dead.

Toward the end of the transplant year, in the spring of 1969, Alice met a patient who would become, as she put it, "my Waterloo."

"We got along exceptionally well until the 49th postoperative day," said Alice, "and then he turned against everybody, even me. He was varyingly euphoric, withdrawn—he refused to eat, or bathe, or walk or cooperate in the least. He became arrogant, haughty, mean, he shot me with silent stares." None of Alice's ploys worked. Her jokes fell flat, her cheerfulness turned sour and stale, her games were thrown against the wall.

Other nurses became reluctant to enter his room. Alice was the only one who attempted to deal with him. "I took the bull by the horns *and* by the tail," she said. "I begged, cajoled, shouted, pleaded, I did everything but get down on my knees beside his bed and make the sign of the cross."

When nothing worked, when for the first time in her life she was totally unable to nurse a patient, Alice decided that perhaps he would improve with a new nurse. Emotionally torn, exhausted, ashamed, she resigned and left the transplant unit. Two days later the patient went into hysterics and had to be tied down. He accused the patient across the hall of forcing Alice out.

For the first time in almost a year there were no longer those telephone calls in the middle of the night from a wife or a daughter, pleading with Alice to hurry back to the hospital because someone had taken a turn for the worse. Alice had always climbed from her bed and driven across town. But upon entering the room, she had seen so many times that her presence could help only the family.

"Patients get a look in their eyes and you know they are lost," she said. "I can't describe it, but any nurse or doctor has seen it. The patients look at you, they focus on you, but they are looking beyond you, thousands of miles and millions of years. . . ."

CHAPTER

13

"I went into the transplant program with great hope," said Jim Nora when it was all over, and when he could look back with passion that had more or less cooled. Nora is a well-made man with hunched shoulders bent from the depth and breadth of his practice. He rose from a lower-class section of Chicago to attend both Harvard and Yale, then to Houston, where he became a prominent pediatric cardiologist with a sideline specialty in genetics, as well as one of the few political liberals in a city whose medical community was overwhelmingly conservative. In the beginning he had shared Cooley's enthusiasm for the new procedure and had zestfully managed the transplants against rejection. "What more noble purpose could there be in medicine than to return dying people to useful life?" he asked himself. But less than five months into the transplant year there began growing a pain within him that he could not deny. "Before we were through," he said, "I was to feel that it was a small-scale crime against humanity. It became a grotesque joke, a game, a game we cannot ever play again."

The disenchantment set in with Cooley's ninth transplant in the blazing August of 1968. He had by then done more transplants than any other surgeon in the world; the hospital had to install security guards to contain the press and keep them from forbidden areas. Jerry Strong had leaned over the operating table one day and said to Cooley during a valve case, "Tell me, Denton, who was the *second* man to fly the Atlantic solo?"

There appeared at St. Luke's that August a beautiful dark-haired five-year-old girl whose heart muscle was so diseased that Cooley's surgery could not repair it. Both she and her parents agreed to a transplant. Their wait was not long; an eight-year-old boy fell from a tree in a Midwestern state, hit his head, and destroyed his brain. He was the son of a college professor. Nora recalled what happened:

"The two sets of parents met in the lobby outside surgery and both were crying. The parents of the girl made plans to share her with the parents of the boy who was giving up his heart. We were readying the child for a transplant and I can remember saying to myself, 'I must do something different, I must not affect her growth'— how naive this sounds now—'I must be careful with the steroids so I will not affect her psyche.' I wanted her to lead a normal life."

Cooley performed a splendid operation and within 24 hours the child was sitting up in bed coloring. But the next day she rejected, and on the eighth day she was dead.

"The euphoria for me was gone," said Nora. "Our first transplants had seemed so hopeful that we thought we had somehow overcome that basic biological rule: the body rejects to protect itself against foreign matter. But we had not overcome the rule. Not at all."

Nora began urging both in his own hospital and in national medical meetings that only transplants of the very best tissue matches be attempted, but he was not heard. Tissue matches between donor and recipient were graded on a scale from A down to D. An A match would be possible only when an identical twin donated his heart to his twin. Of Cooley's transplants, only one tissue match was graded a C-plus. Seven were graded C, four were C-minus, and eight were D. "Perhaps we should do only one or two transplants a year, but we could make sure that they had a better chance to work," Nora said. Bob Leachman was a powerful senior voice against him. "If we're going to be in this game," said the older cardiologist, "then we're going to need to do enough transplants to make the experiment valid, to determine if it is valid clinical therapy. If we only do five or six, we could get bombed either way. You could have six bad ones or six lucky ones and you'd never really know."

When the pattern of rejection had become a familiar one, Nora, distraught, went to Cooley and in a dramatic confrontation begged him to stop. "At least wait until the matches become better," he pleaded. The surgeon was preparing a new transplant. "This is not a good candidate," said Nora.

"But I've promised the family," Nora remembered Cooley saying. It seemed almost an evangelical laying-on-of-hands. It seemed almost God guiding a scalpel. If a borrowed heart could be kept in place by the surgeon's skill—and by his faith in that skill—then none of Cooley's people would have died.

Disenchantment spread. Don Rochelle was attending a medical meeting in New York when he received a telephone call from the hospital in Houston. After a long and moving struggle for life, one of the transplants had died. Rochelle put down the phone and was near tears. He told his wife, who, on hearing the news, became ill. Both had been especially close to the patient. Rochelle located Cooley at the meeting playing string bass with the Heartbeats, a band composed largely of Houston heart doctors, which is well known in the medical world. When the music was over, Rochelle whispered the saddening report. Cooley shook his head and excused himself to attend a reception. Rochelle had been invited to the same party but he was too overcome to attend.

"Denton was disturbed by the deaths, sure," said one member of his team, "but he didn't lose much sleep over them. He gave them the most beautiful surgery in the world. It was not the surgeon's fault that the patient died."

Nora tried to point out that two of America's most distinguished heart surgeons, John Kirklin of Alabama and Dwight McGoon of the Mayo Clinic did not attempt a single transplant. Jim Hardy of Mississippi did but one. Only two were attempted in Russia. Cooley remained convinced of the procedure's validity.

For a time, Cooley even felt that variations on the theme were perhaps possible. One such departure from the norm—if indeed there was a norm to heart transplantation—turned into a bizarre and dark comedy.

When a donor heart could not be found for a dying patient who needed one, Cooley elected to take a ram's heart and implant it. The animal heart shriveled and rejected immediately as the human lay on the operating table. In anticipation of possible trouble, a large pig had been brought to Animal House, a small metal-walled laboratory next door to the main hospital. A pig's heart is similar in physiology to a human heart. Word was quickly telephoned to a surgical team standing by there to prepare the pig—the ram's heart had failed. The unwilling animal was chased about the room, caught, and strapped to the table. He was given anesthesia. He went out, then woke up squealing, fighting to break the straps that contained him. An anesthesiologist was called to bring a more powerful drug. Meanwhile, on the third floor operating room of St. Luke's, the Cooley team was trying to keep the human patient alive. Finally too much time passed and Cooley cancelled the procedure. He pronounced his human patient dead before the pig's heart could be tried.

"A certain amount of naïveté can be forgiven," said Nora, "because, after all, the transplantation business was so new, so unknown. But what destroyed it in my opinion was our continuing to do them after so many failures. It was an example of dehumanization by technology."

Nora remembers thinking as he drove to the hospital in the middle of some night to cope with yet another new crisis, "This is symbolic of everything wrong in our world. Fill in the blank, fill in any abuse you want—pollution, Vietnam, bureaucracy—the mechanics of that abuse are comparable with what we are doing."

"There should be a 'Ballad of Leo Boyd,' " said one of the nurses who watched over him during the sixteen months of pain and crisis. "Few men have ever gone through what he did." I saw Boyd only once. It was toward the end of his ordeal and he must have known it, or wished for it. He was sitting up in bed and his skin was the color of old ivory. He was a museum-piece man, his cheeks artificially puffed from the drugs. I did not speak to him except to nod encouragingly, and he returned my hope for him with an almost papal movement of his right hand, a benediction from a transplant.

Jim Nora could no longer bear to even enter his room and had asked Don Rochelle and the others to care for Boyd. "He came to us a magnificent-looking man with great arm muscles," said Nora. "I could not bear to look at his face and see what we had done to this strong, proud man. . . ."

Boyd was born in the tiny Canadian village of Stratfordville in Ontario province. It had 500 people or so when Boyd was a child and most were involved in the harvesting and curing of bright leaf tobacco. Boyd's parents and people were masons who built saw mills, silos, and factories for tobacco processing. Once in a baseball game with a rival village, Boyd's father offered him a dollar for each home run. He hit four in four times at bat and collected four dollars from his proud but astonished father. Boyd had two brothers, both of whom were boisterous outdoor kids. One threw Boyd into a creek, where he hit his head on a stone and almost drowned. The other boxed with him and knocked him down so often that he became angry and learned the way of the gloves and began winning trophies by the time he was fourteen. Boyd became a strapping youth of six feet plus, with dark hair, hazel eyes, powerful arms and legs with muscles that rippled and veins that stood out like rope on a package. In the Canadian army during World War II, he took judo and after but a few lessons was taunted to climb into the ring with a burly teacher. Boyd slammed him to the mat and almost broke the man's back.

Rather than the masonry trade of his family, Boyd chose railroading and in 26 years on the New York Central, advanced from brakeman to conductor to yardmaster. He was not a man to be kept indoors, for he had a quick temper that flared and died; it rarely flashed when he was hunting birds on the plains near his home or moose at North Bay or casting in the pools below Niagara Falls for perch, or bass, or—his lifelong hope—a muskie. At the age of 42 he took up bowling, became an expert, and scored over 200 in every match. He smoked a pack of Camels every day, and took but an occasional drink after bowling or at weddings. He had two daughters and seven granddaughters and a slender, pretty, hard-working wife named Ilene, who adored him.

On an early autumn morning in 1965 Boyd slept late because he was on the 11 A.M. to 7 P.M. shift. He rose, washed his hair, had coffee, and dressed for work. He went to the garage of their home in Niagara Falls, Canada, and Ilene remembers hearing some muffled noises. The ensuing silence worried her. She walked down the long hall of the house and saw her husband sitting on their bed, his face a purple color.

"I've got the worst pains in my chest," he said. "Must be indigestion."

"But you didn't eat any breakfast and nothing special last night. Leo, lay down."

He obeyed and fell backward, rubbing his left arm.

"Leo, honey, have you got pains in your arm?"

"Yes. All up and down."

Ilene started to back hurriedly out of the room. "I'm calling the doctor," she said.

"Oh, don't do that, hon. It'll pass. I'm due at work."

"Leo, I'm scared." A neighbor had suffered similar pains in his arms while sitting in a lawn chair. He had died before he reached the hospital.

Ilene called for an ambulance, which delivered Boyd to Niagara Falls General Hospital. He had suffered a whopping infarct and was hospitalized for seven weeks. "It was a frightening experience for him," remembered Ilene. "He didn't understand why it had happened to him. But he was a good patient. . . . He would always be a good patient."

Boyd asked his doctor why he had suffered a heart attack. The doctor drew a picture of a pipe rusting inside with little particles flaking off and building up until the pipe occludes and when the fluids can no longer pass through the pipe, it ruptures.

For the first time in his active life, Boyd had to stay indoors and grouch for six months of semi-invalidity. He was a prisoner of blood thinners and digitalis and nitro tablets. He won permission to return to work and seemed restored to a normal life except for rare flashes of anginal pain. In September, 1966, Boyd and Ilene drove to Kentucky for the funeral of a relative and upon arriving back in Niagara Falls, Boyd crumpled to the floor with a second heart attack. Another seven weeks in the hospital, followed by months of terrible pains in his back, neck and head. "I'm going out of my mind with this pain," he told Ilene. He would stuff himself with tranquilizers and pain pills and prowl the house at night. Once he fell asleep in a certain chair and became fond of it. The family dachshund, Gretel, was not allowed near that chair. When Boyd discovered her in it one day he picked up the squealing animal and yelled that he was going to kill her. Ilene smuggled the dog out of the house, gave it away, and interested Boyd in tending to tropical fish, more obedient pets.

On an evening in 1966, Boyd went to sleep after Ilene had given him a shot of Demerol, as she had learned to do. "When they first told me I would have to learn to give the shots," remembered Ilene, "I said I couldn't possibly do that . . . but one learns."

Ilene herself was stricken with pneumonia and on this night she lay beside her drugged husband. When the Demerol wore off, Boyd roused himself and begged for another shot. Ilene refused. He began to rage for more pain killer. Ilene insisted she had to follow the regimen laid down by the doctors. Boyd got up and said he was going to walk about the house and try to make the pain go away.

He was gone such a long time that Ilene got up and began to search for him. She discovered him on the couch in the living room, rolling on it, tossing his body from one end to another, crying out, his face contorted in agony. Then he rolled off the couch and onto the floor. "I had never seen a man in such pain before," said Ilene. She called a doctor, who came and, after a rapid examination, said it might be a gall stone. "I don't think it is another heart attack," he said. But at the hospital, the EKG showed a third infarction had destroyed part of Boyd's heart. It was, in fact, his most severe heart attack to date, and during the night his heart arrested. A team resuscitated him, and Ilene was called at home and told to be at the hospital by eight the next morning and to make up some excuse so as not to worry her husband. He was, they said, desperately ill.

Boyd was in an oxygen tent and frowned at seeing his wife so early. "What are you doing here at this hour?"

"I was going downtown shopping," Ilene lied. "They have sales on and I wanted to be there when they opened the doors. . . . So I thought I'd come here first."

"I see. . . ." He was suspicious.

"How are things?" she asked.

"Something bad is wrong. . . ." Boyd was so gray and weakened from the attack that Ilene had to rush from the room. Outside, the doctor said, "Leo cannot possibly live until night. I think you should gather your family to the hospital."

An hour later his heart went into fibrillation but the electric paddles jolted it with current enough to send it back to a fairly normal rhythm. When Ilene saw him later that afternoon, there were burn marks on his chest. But he was alive.

Boyd's life became a grotesque carousel spinning from hospitals to home to doctors' offices, from new drugs to old ones, to increased dosages, to EKG machines, to sentences of doom, to scenes of horror in the living room when he would shriek his fury at Ilene because she would not quiet him with the medication she kept hidden. One doctor suggested that he go to Toronto General, where a bold surgeon might attempt an open-heart procedure. Boyd was elated at the possibility. But the EKGS and cardiograms were far too pessimistic for surgery. "From your studies, we feel you would not have one chance in a million," they said. "A man with a weaker body than yours would already be dead. There is nothing we can do surgically. We're going to put you on medication and, hopefully, strengthen your heart. Come back in six months and we will examine it again."

Boyd's hopes crumpled. He felt he was beyond hope. He went home in despair with thirteen new drugs to take every day. Ilene chattered gaily beside him, but in her mind was ringing the surgeon's report: one branch of Boyd's left coronary artery was 90 percent blocked, a second branch, 30 percent, and the right, 70 percent.

He would yell at Ilene for more Demerol. "What's the difference in giving it to me now or in an hour and a half from now? . . . Woman, I'm dying from pain!" The scenes became such that Ilene felt her sanity was leaving her. She tried to work at a drugstore and slip away in the afternoon to nurse Boyd and he would be, more likely than not, half-conscious and delirious. "It was in and out of the hospital, in and out of the hospital. . . . One Saturday morning we brought him home, and took him back the same night. . . . I called Toronto and said that even though the six months were not up, couldn't we come back and see if anything could be done? The surgeon there agreed. Leo went in for six weeks of tests. I was trying to save money so I was staying with my sister 85 miles from the hospital and commuting to Toronto with Leo's railroad pass. . . . One night he called me and fairly shouted with happiness, 'Come early tomorrow morning! Come extra early! They're going to operate!'"

Ilene rushed to the hospital by dawn and into her husband's room.

She found him curled into a tight ball, facing the wall, his face streaked with tears. "They're not going to do it," he said. "They're sending me home to die."

They waited for death. Boyd took his medicine. Ilene drugged him to erase the pain and bring the sleep. Sometimes she would drive him to Niagara Falls and park and they would look at the happy, beautiful youngsters in yellow slickers, promenading about the mist. Leo Boyd was only 48, but he was an old man. And tired. And deathly sick.

When Boyd picked up the paper in early December, 1967, and read the headline from Capetown, South Africa, he cried for Ilene to come to his bed. "There may be hope for me," he said, thrusting the paper at her. He followed the case hourly, by radio, by newspaper. Ilene was glad for something to occupy his interest. When Blaiberg was transplanted and seemed to be recovering, Boyd asked his doctor in Niagara Falls to explain the transplant procedure. "We may have to send you to South Africa, Leo," said the doctor.

"I'm just about ready to go," he replied.

A few weeks later, Ilene took Boyd to a larger hospital in London, Ontario. They sat in the waiting room for hours, Boyd's breathing echoing through the room like an iron lung. A doctor finally examined him and said his heart would not last the night. "We have heard that so many times," snapped Ilene. "He will not die if you can just find the time to take care of him."

A general practitioner, a Dr. Lamont, came into Boyd's room and said, "I think you should consider a transplant. What would you think of that?"

"There's not much to think about," said Boyd. "Where could I go?"

"Cooley is doing them in Houston, and Grondin in Montreal."

"I'd rather go to Houston. Neither my wife nor me care much for French Canadians."

"Then I take it you want to go for broke in Texas?"

"Is there another choice?"

"Cooley has done five or six. He appears to be the world leader."

"Then he is the lesser of all the evils," said Boyd. "See if he will take me."

Lamont called Cooley and described the case. Cooley said, "Send him down immediately." It was the Thursday before Labor Day, 1968. Boyd had been sick for so many years and had been in and out of so many hospitals that Ilene had lost count. There was a last-minute snarl when no commercial airline would take Boyd because he required oxygen, and it was considered a peril to other passengers. Ilene discovered a private air ambulance would cost $1,350. She had that much saved up, but if she spent it, she would be penniless for the expected long stay in Houston. Their daughter Carolyn called a radio-TV station, which broadcast the need for money and/or a plane. Within ten minutes the money was donated. The flight took ten hours with two doctors on board to give Boyd medication and watch his heart rate.

Ilene and Boyd walked into St. Luke's at 7 P.M. on a Saturday night. Leo thought there would be a committee to greet him, that a heart would be waiting for him. Instead a nurse showed him to Room 301, immediately beside two swinging doors to a foyer. "Every time the swinging door opened," said Ilene, "Leo thought they were coming for him."

He waited eleven weeks before they came for him.

Boyd was under oxygen for most of the eleven weeks. Ilene remembers lying awake night after night in her motel room across from the hospital, waiting for the ambulance cry that would mean a new heart was coming for her husband. One of the Canadian doctors had given him six months to live, and that sentence was used up. "Leo felt he was living on borrowed time," said Ilene. "Every time he heard a siren, he would straighten his shoulders and say, 'This must be it.'"

He was not the only one in such poignant suspense. The "waiters" formed an informal club to exchange news and rumors. A chief topic was the scarcity of donor hearts. By November 1, Cooley had done but two transplants since the middle of August. "It could be that people are tired of the idea of transplants," said Cooley at the time, "that public opinion has swung against them. I certainly have not lost interest." Cooley popped into the waiters' room, if they were sick enough for hospitalization, about twice a week to assure them that the search was still on for usable hearts. Ilene remembered that several of the waiters grew tired of the ordeal, or ran out of money, and left the city. Some died in their beds when their hearts simply stopped. One Flushing, New York, woman was so depressed by the deaths of Everett Thomas and Louie Fierro that she changed her mind about wanting a transplant and returned to New York. "I'll take my chances living with my family," she said. "In Houston I cry all the time like a hysterical child. I didn't fear the operation, but I was so lonely."

"We gossiped together and prayed together," said Ilene. "We were all here for the same thing. Nothing else was on anybody's mind."

When Cooley did transplants on November 5 and again on November 9, a wave of envy swept through the waiters. "We were all terribly jealous," said Ilene.

On a Friday in mid-November, Boyd was depressed. He had heard through the grapevine that George DuBord, a San Antonio contractor, had rejected during the night and was back at the hospital. There was little that was secret about the new hearts. If one coughed, the echo was heard in every waiter's room.

Ilene was leaving to attend a party in honor of the waiting wives. Boyd asked her to bring him a piece of cake. The next morning, Ilene entered the now familiar room with a paper napkin in her hand. Her husband looked strangely exhilarated, as if he were trying to keep a secret. "Hi, honey, here's your cake," Ilene began.

"I think you'd better eat it yourself if it won't keep, because they aren't letting me have any breakfast today."

"Why?" Ilene tried to keep her voice calm.

"I think. . . ." Boyd would not finish the sentence, almost as an actor does not like to talk of a part before he gets it.

"Is there a donor, Leo?"

"There's one coming in. . . ."

The rest of the Saturday was, as Ilene remembers it, "nerve ends." Boyd was only one of three candidates being considered for the heart, if and when it arrived. It was being flown in from some Western state. Moreover, it was cloudy and rainy. Could planes even land? Cooley was rumored out of town. Would somebody else do the transplant? No, they said, Cooley had been located. He would come back if the heart looked good. . . .

The tension, Ilene said, was "unbearable." Boyd was happy but jumpy, "more nervous of the possibility of *not* getting the heart than of getting it. Our kids had had their bags packed and ready to fly down ever since we came to Houston," she said. "But I didn't want to call them unless the transplant was really going to take place. We would not find out for sure until minutes before the opera-

tion. One of the doctors came in and I said, 'Is it going to be Leo?'
He shook his head and said he was not positive. 'Well,' I said, 'How
positive are you?' 'About 95 percent. Give me five more minutes.' "
Ilene rushed to the telephone to call her children. She barely had
time to kiss Boyd good-bye before he went to surgery.

In the surgical waiting room during the transplant operation, Ilene
brushed past a weary, unshaven doctor from Yuma, Arizona. She did
not learn for several days the incredible story of how this man had
brought Boyd a new heart.

Maria Acosta was seven months' pregnant when she fell uncon-
scious in her home in the small town of San Luis, Mexico, near the
Arizona border. She was rushed across the border to Yuma's Park-
view Baptist Methodist, where an obstetrician, Dr. Gerold Gordon,
measured massive brain hemorrhage. The EEG waves were flat, her
eyes did not respond. While she was being examined, her heart arrested. She could not have been more dead.

Gordon delivered Maria of the new life growing within her, and
the baby had a slim chance at survival. The doctor felt that Maria
had still more life to give—her heart, provided he could win permission to use it. She had a common-law husband who was told through
an interpreter what Gordon proposed. Confused, frightened, the
man refused in tears. Gordon then learned that Maria's mother and a
grown daughter lived but 25 miles on the other side of the Mexican
border and, blood kin being more binding than common law, their
signature would probably be more legal. The doctor raced his car
across the border and into the small town. With a passionate speech
about the highest gift of all, the gift of life, Gordon waited for it to
be translated. The mother and daughter hesitated. He promised that
if the heart could not be used, he would bury Maria as soon as it
stopped beating. Permission was won; the mother signed the hastily
dictated form with an "X," witnessed by the older daughter. Gordon
thanked them deeply and said there would be no hospital bill or doctor's fee for Maria.

Maria Acosta's heart was still beating, the ventilator breathing for
her and drugs keeping her pressure at a satisfactory level. In his absence, Gordon's nurse had run tests and discovered that Maria's

blood type was O, universal, her Rh factor was plus, there was a lack of oxygen in the heart but no massive damage. It was a promising heart for transplantation.

Gordon called Houston and asked for Cooley. He was not there; Grady Hallman took the telephone. The heart sounded highly usable but could Gordon get it to Houston? He would try. For six hours Gordon battled military red tape before he finally got someone to produce a Navy jet trainer. It took off at 9:30 P.M. with Gordon, his nurse, and the stretcher containing Maria wedged into the tiny compartment. Gordon told Phoenix journalist Earl Zarbin of the trip: The stretcher had to be placed on top of the oxygen tank, the respirator leaned against another tank, the intravenous bottles hung like clothes on a washline. The high-altitude flight in the nonpressurized craft interfered with the intravenous drip and the nurse had to hold the bottles in her hand and force the fluids into Maria's arm. When the plane approached Houston, Gordon was horrified to learn that the coastal city was covered with fog and landing was impossible. The pilot made arrangements to put down in San Antonio, 200 miles away, and radioed ahead for an ambulance.

An Air Force ambulance screamed through the dawn fog toward Houston at speeds from 80 to 100 miles per hour. The respirator breathing for Maria was coming apart and Gordon held it together with his hands. Oxygen tanks had come loose and were banging about like barn doors in a storm, bruising everyone they hit. Bottles broke and sloshed liquids. Maria's thoracic cavity was filling with fluid, her heart was skipping beats. Gordon fantasized it would collapse and stop in grotesque irony on the very doorsteps of the hospital. When the ambulance entered the city, no one in it knew where St. Luke's Hospital was nor did any of the people they stopped. Somehow an escort from the police materialized and led them through the fog to the hospital. The emergency flight that had begun at 9:30 the night before was over at 8 A.M.

Someone asked Gordon about the legality of bringing a Mexican national across state lines to Houston for an operation to remove her heart and give it to a man from Canada.

"I imagine I must have broken six laws," said Gordon, "But we'll worry about that later. . . ."

Ilene went to the chapel, where she was surrounded by friends, chaplains, a waiter or two, a newspaper reporter. She prayed almost continuously for five hours. In the late afternoon Cooley came in with a tense face; he was still in his scrub suit and there were spots of blood on it. He had obviously hurried from surgery with the news. Ilene thought the world would turn upside down before he spoke. "Everything seems to be fine," he said, bending his mouth into a smile. He seemed exceptionally worn. "The heart started on its own, it didn't even require a shock. His pressure's about 130. I think he's already conscious. He seems to know us. . . ."

At 6 A.M. the next morning, Ilene and her daughters were permitted to enter the operating room still being used for recovery. Alice Nye had prepared the women for how Leo Boyd would look—the tubes, the bottles, the wires, the yellow-orange chest, the smell of mingling drugs. But it was still a shock to see the strong railroad man in such circumstances. Ilene bent forward and kissed him gently.

"I felt like the burden of the world had been lifted from me," she said later that day. "Those eleven weeks here, those years in all the hospitals, the hell is over. . . ." Ilene spent the rest of the day praying her gratitude.

Because his recovery seemed so routine and because there was no hint of rejection, Boyd was moved into Alice's transplant unit on the first postoperative day. On the second day he stood beside his bed. Ilene put on masks, gown, hat, and boots and went to her husband. They looked at each other for a few moments. Boyd became emotional and wept. Ilene's mask could not hide her tears.

"Well, I finally got it, honey. . . ." Boyd gestured toward the enormous bandage at his breast.

"And you're doing just fine. . . . Everything is going to be just fine, Leo. Just like you always knew it would."

Boyd lived for sixteen months but he never left the hospital for more than a few hours. He never returned to his beloved Canada. No sooner was one crisis over than another took its place. The supreme technology and knowledge of the Cooley team kept him alive, but the life they sustained within him was a cruel one.

For three months he did well. He walked about his room, strolled masked down the corridors, proud of the circulation provided from the Mexican woman's heart. He asked to go home, but Nora and Rochelle wanted him to stay in the hospital. They were alarmed at the sudden deaths of Thomas and Fierro and DuBord; Boyd was Cooley's fifteenth transplant and only five were still alive.

Bursitis developed in Boyd's right arm and shoulder. It became so painful that he could not lift his arm from the bed. One morning he told Ilene, "Honey, I think it's crossing over to the left." And that night he could lift neither arm. The previous night he had heard the emergency cart with the bottles clanging and clattering down the hall to the room of another transplant, and the transplant had died. It was, Boyd told his wife, like an executioner coming to get the condemned man. He begged Alice to let him sleep in another part of the hospital; he feared to be alone in the transplant unit with his arms useless beside him. Alice joked and made him laugh and he passed the night fitfully.

The bursitis went away and a rejection episode set in, the first. Boyd could not eat, then would not eat. He was nauseated continually but could not vomit. Ilene said, "I kept telling myself this wasn't happening. I told Leo it was some little virus so often that I almost believed it myself. I don't think he realized the heart was being rejected."

After a month, when all the familiar symptoms of rejection would not go away, Rochelle took Ilene aside and said it would be best to gather the family. Ilene made up a story to fool her husband about the girls flying down to Houston, a pathetic story that they had saved their baby-sitting money and were coming to surprise him.

But he did not die. He did not die so many times that Ilene—and the doctors—began to feel he was somehow invincible. "He fought so hard," said Ilene. "He obeyed all the orders, he took his blowing machine twice a day, he put on the mist mask, which a lot of the others refused. Leo used it every day of his new life. . . ."

He was just getting over his first rejection episode when he was stricken with meningitis. Rochelle explained to Ilene that every human being carries a little meningitis around in his body, but Boyd's resistance from the immunosuppressive drugs was so low that he was unable to fight it. When a month of meningitis was over, he was starting to walk around his room again when one day, standing beside his bed, his knees buckled, he fell to the floor and cracked a vertebra. Bone softening is a common complication of long-term steroids. For six weeks he was bedridden with a back brace. A cyst coincidentally appeared behind his knee cap. The doctors drained fluid collected there and attached a leg brace in addition to the back brace.

There were good hours. There was a first anniversary (one year with his new heart) party with a red heart cake and a new suit, which Boyd happily got into to pose for pictures. There were always the newspaper reporters and he enjoyed answering their questions and clipping out his name. He spent a few weekends at Ilene's apartment near the hospital, where she happily cooked him ham hocks and navy beans, his favorite dish. He even gamely answered the psychiatrist's questions, normally replying, somewhat mischievously, "a naked woman," when asked what a Rorschach ink blob looked like to him. There was but a brief two-day period of confusion and disorientation. Boyd insisted that he had won a Sweepstakes race and was upset that Ilene could not find the huge check in his dresser drawer. "I know it's there, honey, keep looking!" he cried, as Ilene rummaged sadly through his things.

"Leo did not have the psychic problems that so many of the others did." said Ilene. "Considering what happened to the others, I am grateful that his mind did not suffer."

For Christmas, 1968, the children and grandchildren came from Canada and New York and there was, as Ilene remembers, a "muted family celebration." A few days later, another rejection episode, a final rejection episode, struck his heart and destroyed his body. Pneumonia smothered him, his kidneys deteriorated, he was forced in the last two weeks of life to urinate through a catheter. Cooley came one night toward the end and took Boyd's hand and gripped it. He studied the x-rays and EKGS and said, "we're not licked yet." Boyd was the last one alive, the last living model of the splendid operation, the ravaged testimony to the grace and daring—and ambition—of the surgeon's hands. On the day before Easter, 1970, Boyd wanted something. He turned his head this way, then that way, he pleaded with his eyes for Ilene to help him. She held her husband in her arms and tried to reach for the Panic Button to bring doctors running. But her sister held her back. "Leo closed his eyes," said Ilene, "Leo was gone."

Rochelle broke. "He cried," said Ilene, "more than I did." Nora was devastated by the death. He wept for the man but he wept as well for the morality of the process. It had cost more than $160,000 to keep Boyd alive. "I couldn't help but think what would happen if we had taken $160,000 and spent it in India on children with yaws," said Nora. "I wondered just what was moral anymore. This was a small corner of my life, I kept telling myself, not successfully, a not very major corner. . . ."

Cooley asked Ilene if she would permit a memorial service for Boyd the next day, Easter morning. None had been held for the other transplants, but then, none had so captured and held the hospital's mind as had Boyd. Ilene agreed. The chapel next day was full. The service was brief, moving. The chaplain spoke of Boyd's courage and of Ilene's. Prayers were held to speed his resurrection on the Easter day. Alice Nye, for the first time since she had begun to nurse the transplanted hearts, cracked, and put her head in her strong hands and cried.

"Leo did it for me, and for the children," said Ilene. "But he also did it for the doctors. He loved them all—Cooley, Rochelle, Nora, Bloodwell. They gave him sixteen months of new life—hard life, yes, but life! He saw a man walk on the moon and he saw his children and grandchildren grow older. Why, he met so many celebrities . . . the King and Queen of Belgium. . . . One day Cooley called and said 'Dress Leo up, Christiaan Barnard wants to see him,' and Leo was so happy and Barnard said, 'You don't even look sick enough to be in the hospital.' . . . Leo's autograph book was full of famous doctors' names. Oh, I think he would go through it all again. . . . He was a man who laughed and joked until there was nothing more to laugh at. . . ."

CHAPTER
14

There was a conspicuous silence at Methodist Hospital in the immediate months after Christiaan Barnard performed his first transplant and startled the world. Mike DeBakey had made an immediate statement of congratulation to the South African surgeon. "He has broken the ice," said DeBakey, when asked by a reporter for his reaction. "It is a real breakthrough in the whole field of heart replacement. It is a great achievement." There were, DeBakey said, at least twenty medical centers in the world where there was skill and knowledge enough to perform transplants. "What we've all been waiting for," he went on, "is the right circumstances—the right donor and the right recipient. Dr. Barnard had the right circumstances and he did it. They took the first step. We will do it, too."

But the months began to pass and across the way at neighboring St. Luke's, Cooley began his program in May. And by mid-summer, 1968, when Cooley had become the man who had done more heart transplants than any surgeon in the world, DeBakey, somewhat uncharacteristically, had not yet moved. He seemed almost reluctant to enter the transplant business. He commented more and more about transplants being but a "way station" on the road to an artificial heart, the road he had been traveling for almost a decade. He called for more federal funds to support the artificial-heart research. "If we mobilized our resources like we do to launch artificial satellites," he said, in the city where science had reached the moon, "say 4 or 5 billion dollars, then we would get the artificial heart much faster." And in speeches and papers, DeBakey urged the need for exceptional caution and judgment from surgical teams before deciding to do heart-transplant surgery.

DeBakey, in the March, 1968, issue of the *Journal of Thoracic and Cardiovascular Surgery*, wrote, "Since the physician can never afford to delay medical treatment until knowledge is complete and risk is entirely removed, he must apply current knowledge cautiously and judiciously, weighing the benefits against the hazards, in his efforts to relieve suffering and cure disease. Continued clinical trials [of transplants] are therefore necessary, but only after the most sober deliberation and most prudent consideration of all present evidence of their potential usefulness and limited scope. The indications for transplantation of the human heart at present must therefore be carefully delineated.

"The competing risks must be thoroughly assessed: application of a procedure, results of which are not completely known, against withholding of a clinical trial that may save the patient's life. Such assessment requires the sagest, most deliberate judgment, based on extensive clinical experience in the cardiovascular field and on the knowledge and skills acquired in the specialized cardiovascular research and transplantation centers of the world."

Despite DeBakey's sensible and cool attitude toward transplants, his staff nonetheless chafed to get into the business. The vast medical and scientific resources of Baylor had begun making their own ALG— the immunosuppressive drug; they had arranged a liaison with Terasaki in Los Angeles for rapid tissue-typing. Moreover, the Fondren-Brown Cardiovascular Center, though not yet fully opened in 1968, had an elaborate area for transplant recovery and postoperative intensive care. Ted Diethrich, George Noon, and several of the residents began practicing transplants on dogs. By August, 1968, the DeBakey team was better prepared than Cooley and his staff were when they had begun transplantations three months earlier.

"We were ready to go," said Ted Diethrich. "In fact, we were raring to go." But it went without saying that it would take a spectacular achievement to catch up to what Cooley was doing with such apparent success across the way. Unknown to DeBakey, Diethrich and his friend John Liddicoat, a surgical resident from Michigan, drew up in their spare time a complicated outline of organizational structure, a plan for an incredible operation or series of operations. It was their audacious idea that a multiple transplant could take place using various organs from the same donor. If conditions were suitable, a donor's heart, lung, and both kidneys could be transplanted into four different people in four different operating rooms at the same time. It would entail breathtaking precision, teamwork, and the talents of almost one hundred medical personnel. But if it could be brought off, it would be an amazing feat.

When the charts had been meticulously prepared, listing in minute detail everything from how many movie photographers were required for each of the four operating rooms down to weekend telephone numbers for standby nurses, Diethrich sent word quietly out through the hospitals of Houston and surrounding areas that he would like to be notified if a promising donor heart turned up.

On the last day of August, 1968, Diethrich was driving down a Houston freeway when he received a squawk on his beeper, the radio paging system used by doctors. He answered the call and was told to get in touch with a nurse at St. Joseph's Hospital. Diethrich was puzzled because St. Joseph's was a hospital in downtown Houston not connected with the Texas Medical Center and a hospital at which he neither operated nor had connections. He turned off the freeway quickly and found a telephone. The nurse at St. Joseph's spoke in a whisper. "We have a girl who has shot herself in the head," she said *sotto voce*. "That's all I know, but if you want to come down you can talk to her doctor."

Diethrich remembers he tried "not to sound excited" as he thanked the nurse and hung up. He telephoned Liddicoat and said, "This is it, I think we're on countdown. Change clothes and meet me at Methodist right away." The two young doctors slipped out of business clothes and into surgical greens with white lab coats—the uniform of office is far more eloquent and persuasive than a blazer and flannel slacks. Arriving at St. Joseph's at 9 P.M., Diethrich found the doctor attending the gunshot victim. "She's a kid about nineteen or twenty, Latin American I think," said the doctor. "She shot herself in the brain. If we shut the respirator off, she's gone."

"What about a heart transplant?" asked Diethrich.

The doctor shook his head. "We've never had a donor here. I simply don't know the procedure."

"First of all," said Diethrich hurriedly. "She has to be pronounced neurologically dead."

"Well, we can do that right now. Just hook up the EEG."

"Second of all," said Diethrich, "we need permission from the next of kin. Who is that?"

"There's a husband, I believe. She'd only been married a few months."

"Where is the husband?"

"I have no idea."

A nurse hovering nearby interrupted cautiously. "The police came by and locked him up. He's in jail."

"Why?" asked Diethrich.

"Perhaps they don't believe it was suicide."

"How much time do you have before the heart would be useless to you?" asked the doctor.

"I don't know for sure," said Diethrich. "There's already a slight decrease in blood pressure." At that moment, Diethrich remembers, he almost cancelled the entire plan. There seemed to be a police-legal snarl—it might take wasted hours to unravel it. "But just as a chance that it might go," said Diethrich, "I called the kidney and lung transplant team leaders at Methodist and told them to stand by."

That night in Methodist Hospital, four patients were waiting for organ transplants. One man with severe emphysema needed a lung, two others—one 50, one 22—wanted new kidneys. Bill Carroll, a factory worker from Scottsdale, Arizona, had come to Methodist for open-heart surgery, but tests had revealed that nothing could be done. Diethrich had suggested a transplant, offering him the services of neighboring St. Luke's and Cooley, or, if he was willing to wait a few days or weeks, the untried capacities of the DeBakey team. Carroll agreed quickly to the transplant and said, "I'll try my luck with you, Ted."

Diethrich drew a vial of blood from the girl who had shot herself—whom we will call Mrs. Gonzalez—and rushed it by messenger to the Baylor laboratories. There the typing and testing could begin while Diethrich sought to see if legally the heart could be used.

Diethrich raced out of St. Joseph's and drove at high speeds the two miles across downtown Houston to the central police station. In the homicide division, an officer was familiar with the case but said, "Doc, I just don't know—or can't tell what happened. We brought the kid in because he was hysterical. He saw his wife at St. Joe's and collapsed. He hasn't quieted down long enough for us to question him."

"Where is he?" asked Diethrich. "May I talk to him?"

The policeman nodded. He took the young surgeon to a small questioning room, a barren place with cold walls, a table, two hard chairs, a coffee can for cigarette butts. The young husband, Raul Gonzalez, confused, sobbing, was brought in and left alone with Diethrich. "I'm Dr. Diethrich," he said, "I've just come from the hospital and your wife is doing very poorly. I don't think she can possibly make it." The youth began screaming; Diethrich cut through bluntly.

"I want to know how it happened. It is very important to know *exactly* how it happened."

Suddenly Raul Gonzalez quieted. He cupped his head in his hands and began to talk. His marriage, he said, had been a stormy one and his wife had become despondent over financial problems. She had threatened suicide four months earlier. On this second night they had been driving down a road when she suddenly produced a gun, put it to her head, and shot herself.

"Right there in the car, sitting beside you?" asked Diethrich, picturing the grisly scene.

The youth nodded and began to cry again.

Diethrich cut through once again. He asked his most important question. "Was it an accident? Or suicide? Or did *you* do it?" If it had been either of the first two, Diethrich felt he could use the girl's heart. But if he suspected that a homicide had taken place, he could not. Already there had been the unpleasant incident over Cooley using the heart of Clarence (Sonny) Nicks. DeBakey and his staff had agreed with the medical examiner's plea not to transplant hearts that might be involved in a murder trial.

"It was suicide, Doctor," said Gonzalez. "She shot herself." His face, his words seemed so convincing that Diethrich believed him. A homicide lieutenant came in and talked privately with the youth. When he was done he spoke with Diethrich in an outer office. "I'll go with suicide," he said. "I'll accept your medical judgment. I'm releasing him in your custody, but we'll still want to talk to him a little more."

On the unsettling drive to St. Joseph's, with Gonzalez sniffling in the back seat, Diethrich brought up the idea of a heart transplant. The youth seemed unable to comprehend what the young doctor was saying; Diethrich dropped it for the time being. In the hour he had been away, all of the girl's relatives had flocked to the hospital and were crowded outside the emergency room where she was being attended. Diethrich tried to find the voice of authority in the family but none rose above the hysteria. The rosary beads were out in the purging rite of grief. Gonzalez demanded to see his wife, and Diethrich unwisely agreed. The moment the youth saw his wife on her medical bier, the breathing machine forcing her chest to rise and fall, the intravenous tubes sending the fluids of false-hope through her useless body, the monitoring machines clicking and chanting about her, he cried, in exultation, "But she's alive! She breathes! Her chest is moving!" Diethrich took him by the arm and led him outside and for more than an hour tried to explain what "neurologically dead" meant, with the family flocked about answering in Spanish and English. The girl's sister and sister-in-law emerged as the most intelligent, rational voices in the family unit and they seemed resigned to the difficult fact that the girl was alive only by the grace of the machines and once their force was shut off, then nothing would be left. They seemed flattered at Diethrich's suggestion that their relative could perhaps give life to a stranger. They persuaded Raul Gonzalez to agree to transfer his wife to Methodist for "further evaluation." Diethrich promised to have another EEG taken there. Gonzalez nodded; in one hour he had learned what brain waves are and how they govern the destiny of the earthly soul.

Convinced that he could win permission from Gonzalez to take not only his wife's heart but a lung and both kidneys as well, Diethrich once again telephoned Methodist and set the plan in action. Calls went out quickly for the four teams—more than 75 people—to report to the hospital in secrecy. In the hour and a half that it took to arrange for the girl's transfer by ambulance from St. Joseph's across town to Methodist, all four of the recipient patients had been prepped, photographed, given antibiotics and ALG, their blood typed. The hospital was swept up in the urgent exhilaration of the event when Ted arrived. A second EEG was taken of the girl's brain by a neurologist not connected with the transplant team and the waves were flat. Diethrich showed the monitor to Gonzalez, who looked at it only briefly before he nodded. He agreed to the doctors using whatever part of his wife they felt necessary. "Her soul is with God," one of the sisters had said earlier, and Gonzalez repeated it now over and over again.

At 11:30 P.M. Diethrich called DeBakey at home and for the first time informed him of what was being prepared at Methodist. DeBakey asked the bare particulars of the case, then wanted to know what any surgeon would: Where would the blood come from in the middle of the night for four sudden major surgeries? "Everything is under control," said Diethrich. "I'm going to the blood bank right now." Between sixteen and twenty pints would have to be found. DeBakey was skeptical as to whether four surgeries could be done. He felt only the heart transplant should be attempted. He had not known of the elaborate battle plan that his junior man had drawn up in the study of his own home.

There were last-minute problems; the hospital's administration wanted a legal officer to check that the permission forms had been properly signed and that a neutral physician had pronounced the donor dead. The medical photography department had difficulty finding enough photographers to staff four operating chambers and the donor's room. DeBakey arrived at 1 A.M. and was impressed enough by the fervor of his staff that he endorsed what was to be attempted.

"We held our breath because DeBakey could have cancelled the whole thing at that point," said one of the junior men. "He walked around to all of the rooms and saw how everybody was working together, how beautifully Ted and John's battle plan was coming off, and he realized a series of four transplants would not only be history, but Something Else!" Moreover, six months had passed since DeBakey had written his plea for caution in heart transplantation, and much had been learned.

At 1:45 A.M. the historic procedures began.

The dead girl was placed in Room 5, Bill Carroll, who would receive the heart was in 4, the lung recipient in 2, the kidney recipients in 6 and 7. Diethrich opened Carroll and removed his diseased heart. He went across to Room 5 and performed a median sternotomy on the donor, removing her heart and saving a piece of pulmonary vein for the atrium and anastomosis (suturing) to Carroll's lung. While Diethrich with DeBakey sewed in the girl's heart, other surgeons went, in turn, to the cadaver in Room 5 and took what they needed —first the lung, then the kidneys. "It could not have gone more smoothly," said Diethrich later. "If we had rehearsed the thing a thousand times, it could not have come off better." One by one the patients were transferred across the elevated corridor that connects Methodist with Fondren-Brown and all were installed in the sterile transplant-recovery suite.

One of the kidney recipients, the 50-year-old man, died of a heart attack one month later. The lung recipient died about the same time. But the young man who received the girl's other kidney not only recovered but married the nurse who cared for him in Intensive Care. Bill Carroll defied what was known of the then infant art of heart transplantation.

When the report came back from Terasaki in Los Angeles the day after Carroll received his heart, it revealed that he and the girl were a D-match, the poorest type on the scale. But he not only tolerated the heart, he regained almost robust health, returned to Phoenix and found an active job as a worker in a sheet-metal factory, resumed his passion for golf and told Diethrich proudly that his marriage was better than it ever had been. He was alive, spectacularly alive more than two and a half years postoperatively when this book was completed. He personified everything the operation should be and do, but so rarely was and did.

The transplanters received one tantalizing clue from studying Carroll's case. All people are either hyper-reactors, meaning their bodies react strongly to something, or, conversely, they are hypo-reactors. Carroll was a hypo-reactor. When foreign protein is in-

jected into a hypo-reactor, his body pays less attention to it. In a
highly sophisticated test, white cells are taken from the blood, grown
in a culture dish, and challenged with foreign protein. Either they
react or do not react. "Perhaps we should transplant only the hypo-
reactors," mused Ted as he elatedly studied Carroll's progress.

Five days after the multiple transplant procedures, the "DeBakey
team," as it would become known in the press, performed their second heart transplant. Their success was considerably less; the patient died on the eighth day.

Their third was the most remarkable of all. Duson Vlaco, a sixteen-
year-old Yugoslavian boy, had been in Methodist for two weeks
while the cardiologists studied him. Shockingly thin, the boy had a
grotesque collection of congenital heart defects. He was born with
an AV commune, meaning that he had a common atrium and ventricle; only one chamber in effect, rather than the four of the normal
heart. Blood sloshed back and forth within the deformed pump fighting to get in and out. The tricuspid and mitral valves were malformed. He had arms and legs like toothpicks and he weighed, upon
arrival, less than sixty pounds. It was an act of enormous pain
merely to gaze upon the boy, much less probe his pitiful body for
the possibility of surgical relief. "He was the sickest human being I
had ever laid eyes on," said Diethrich.

On the evening of September 15, 1968, Duson lay in his hospital bed half-propped up because his lungs were so filled with edema
that fluid bubbled up and spilled from his lips. Had he been flat on
his back he would have drowned in his own juices. The decision
already had been made that there was nothing to be done surgically.
The heart doctors were trying to deplete the fluid so Duson could
fly back to Yugoslavia and die on his native soil. At 11 P.M. Diethrich was called to the boy's room because he seemed to be in terminal
failure. The look of death was in his eyes, his mother sat helplessly
beside her only child. Neither she nor the boy spoke English and
they depended upon a Yugoslavian cardiologist who had accompanied them to translate. Mrs. Vlaco stood up in despair when
Diethrich entered the room. He made a brief examination of the boy
and took her to a corner where he talked quietly. "I don't think he
will last until morning," he said. The translator hesitated, then repeated. Mrs. Vlaco threw her hand to her face at the condemning

sentence. There was, Diethrich said, a patient who had been brought a few hours earlier to neurological intensive care. He had suffered pancreatis and cardiac arrest but had been resuscitated. His brain was dead. His family had agreed to donating his heart to anyone who needed one.

If Duson and his mother wanted, Diethrich told the Yugoslavian doctor, he would attempt a transplant as "an emergency, a desperate act." No tissue typing had been done on the boy, nor would there be time. His condition was so grave and his body so massively deteriorated by the malfunctioning heart that the odds were overwhelmingly against success. The proposition was put to the mother. She shook her head almost immediately. "No," she said in her native language, "we heard about transplants before we came to Houston but neither Duson nor I want it." "I understand your point of view," the surgeon said, "but we don't have another thing to offer him. We'll do the very best we can with medicines, but it's a mechanical problem within his heart and we just can't fix it." Diethrich turned and walked from the room. No sooner was he in the corridor when the broken voice of the mother stopped him.

"Doctor! Doctor! Please!" she cried in English. Her hands were outstretched. The Yugoslavian cardiologist spoke for her. "She wants the transplant. She wants her son saved."

The transplant began within an hour. The anesthesiologist, who had to put the boy to sleep in a sitting-up position because of the pulmonary edema said, "Ted, you've lost your mind." Diethrich resisted a shudder himself as he sliced into the taut chest and encountered the huge, flaccid heart. This is what the operation is all about, he said to himself. This is a dying patient. There is nothing else for him. If there is a justification for heart transplantation, it is lying before me on this table.

Within two weeks, Duson was greedily taking food. Within four weeks he was chattering in English. Quickly he was up and about the hospital. He learned to play the guitar and serenaded the nurses. He laughed for the first time in years. He got a part-time job helping feed the dogs and experimental animals in the Baylor laboratories. He shook Diethrich's hand hard when he flew back to Yugoslavia. There he formed a rock-and-roll band and began making records. He wrote Diethrich several months later that his song, written in honor of the Houston-based astronauts, was rapidly climbing up the Yugoslavian pop charts.

The DeBakey team did all in all twelve transplants, and by the beginning of summer, 1971, both Bill Carroll and Duson Vlaco were still very much alive. Diethrich felt the results were, in fact, better than the statistics. "We had two patients die from infection, from colon problems not related to the heart," he said. "The transplanted hearts were working fine. We had one patient in whom the donor heart failed. We had another who died of a cerebral embolus, a clot to the brain. It could have happened to anybody. The statistics are not really as bad as they sound on the surface. I truly believe this can be a useful operation. There are two witnesses, one in Phoenix, one in Belgrade, who will testify to it."

The legitimacy of the surgeon in the world of medicine—the supreme academic moment of his long ascent from barber to eminence—was ensured when Michael E. DeBakey was installed as president and chief executive officer of the Baylor College of Medicine in May, 1968, about the time that Denton Cooley was beginning his transplant program. No one could remember if a surgeon had ever become president of a major medical school. Nor could anyone understand why DeBakey would want the job; his curriculum vitae was already eighteen closely printed pages long.

There had been two immediate presidents of Baylor who had feuded with the board of trustees. They had left with the school in financial distress. One Houston doctor remarked, "Baylor was broke, there was practically no fiscal program. It was heading downhill fast. DeBakey volunteered to take over as a kind of interim chief executive to get the school back on its feet. Nobody in Houston medicine had the glamorous image he did, he could raise money, he could attract great teachers. But there was a fight from those who did not want him to take over as president. They knew how much work he already had, and they wanted a full-time president. Mike beat them down, he always wins. He wanted to be president and he became president." Leachman had once remarked as to what drove the Cooleys and the DeBakeys of the world: "They seek to leave bigger footprints than anybody else." DeBakey's were now gigantic. He had operated on royalty, he had dazzled the scientific world with his surgery, his name was a household word, and now he was president of one of America's leading medical schools. Someday he would crown his career with the perfection of an artificial heart.

One of his first steps as president of Baylor was to sever the school from its parent institution, Baylor University in Waco, Texas, a conservative Baptist school whose leaders once fired the noted theatrical director Paul Baker from its faculty because he refused to delete the profanity from a Eugene O'Neill play.

Much of 1968 was spent by DeBakey in establishing a fiscal policy for the now independent medical school. He sought out private and public money. Those who previously had difficulty in obtaining the DeBakey ear now complained that it took weeks instead of days before he would return a telephone call, much less grant an appointment—if at all. One who was exceptionally frustrated was Dr. Domingo Liotta, the surgeon researcher who had been laboring for five long years in the secluded laboratories of Baylor, building and testing and discarding and starting again with hundreds of intricate plastic and metal parts, hoping to be the first man in history to develop, under DeBakey's sponsorship, an artificial heart. His work had received dramatic impetus with the wave of human heart transplantations dominating the press. And because the human hearts were not being tolerated as well as had been expected, the mechanical one loomed all the more paramount. DeBakey had many times predicted the coming of the artificial heart in speeches before medical meetings and congressional committees. He told of the great promise that it held. In 1964, DeBakey had made a flat prediction that the artificial heart would be ready for implantation in a human within three to five years. But in mid-1968 he upped that another five. Liotta was more optimistic. By September, 1968, he and his associates had developed a prototype, which seemed to hold great promise. But when Liotta sought to convince DeBakey of this, he was turned away. Impatience is a disease that strikes every man at least one moment of his life, and it found fertile ground in Houston. Liotta felt he stood on the threshhold of greatness, but that his way was being blocked by the most famous—and often exasperating—surgeon in America. "Every time

Domingo finally got through to Mike to urge that more attention be paid to the artificial heart," said one Houston doctor, "he would be told to get back down to the laboratory and continue his work. Mike keeps his eye on people and their work in his own way. But there were weeks, sometimes months, when Liotta couldn't get through to Mike at all. He began to feel DeBakey was simply not interested in the artificial heart."

There was to be an alternative. Liotta had long admired Denton Cooley. When he had first come to Houston in 1961 and was still not comfortable in English, Liotta had found Cooley to be kind to him. The Texan had sponsored the Latin's candidacy for a national scientific association. They had remained friends over the years, Cooley appreciating Liotta's skill in the research labs, Liotta frankly spellbound by Cooley's dash in the surgical suites. In early December of 1968, the two doctors met in private. Liotta expressed his anguish over what he felt was difficulty in getting DeBakey to move toward a clinical test of the artificial heart. Cooley nodded in sympathy. He knew DeBakey well. When their conversation was done, they made a secret pact that would bring the transplant year in Houston to an explosive climax, one that would wrench the world of medicine, and strip bare the ambition and jealousies and furies of those who work in the human heart.

In the first days of April, 1969, there emerged these facts:

1. On April 4, Denton Cooley, with Domingo Liotta at his side, became the first surgeon in history to implant an artificial heart into a patient, Haskell Karp, a 47-year-old printing estimator from Illinois.

2. Cooley, with Mrs. Karp beside him, went on television and radio the next day to announce the historic operation, to explain that it was a desperate, stop-gap measure because no human donor heart had been available, and to appeal nationally for such a human heart, which could be substituted for the plastic and metal one— powered by a huge, freezer-sized console standing beside Karp's bed.

3. Karp lived for 63 hours with the artificial device before it was removed in favor of a donor heart taken from a 40-year-old woman,

whose body had been flown by chartered jet from Massachusetts in answer to the Cooley appeal.

4. Karp died about twenty hours later.

The Karp affair became the Chinese box of medicine, a complex puzzle of ethics and science wrapped deep within the passions of men, not to be fully unraveled by committees and testimony. De-Bakey first heard of the operation the morning after, when he walked into a Washington, D.C. meeting of the National Heart Institute, from whom he had received grants to develop the artificial heart. Never a man with time to read the newspapers or listen to the radio, he had neither seen nor heard Mrs. Karp's appeal for a human heart. The men at the Washington meeting crowded around DeBakey and pressed him for particulars of the breakthrough, if there had been a breakthrough.

Cooley was, after all, a member of the Baylor faculty and De-Bakey was its president. Cooley had been linked with DeBakey in the medical world's mind for almost two decades. Surely DeBakey would know what had happened the night before at the hospital next door to him. But DeBakey knew nothing. He was more surprised than any man in the room. How ironic, in fact, how cruel, that the rug should be pulled in the presence of his peers. One doctor said that DeBakey's face went white with rage.

As soon as he got back to Houston, DeBakey immediately launched a private investigation. The first thing he learned was that Domingo Liotta had been serving two masters—working for some four months not only for Mike DeBakey, but in secret for Denton Cooley as well. He was serving both surgeons on the same Herculean task—developing the artificial heart.

The second thing DeBakey discovered was that the device implanted in Haskell Karp looked amazingly like the very one Mike DeBakey knew was being developed in his own laboratories. "They used the exact same heart," he said when he looked at the drawing St. Luke's had released to the press. Months later, in conversation with a friend, DeBakey brandished the drawing and said, "Look! They weren't even clever enough to make it look different!"

Cooley's immediate answer was that Liotta had worked for him privately, on nights and during weekends, and that the heart they developed, with some $20,000 of Cooley's money, was independent from the one that DeBakey was producing. Moreover, Cooley pointed out, he was a member of the Baylor faculty, a full professor of surgery, and was entitled to use the research knowledge that flowed from the school's laboratories. What was research for in medicine, if not to serve the clinician?

Liotta was asked by a reporter how he could conscientiously work for two men on the same project. "It's a sticky thing and I don't think it would be right to put it in the press." As to the heart, he hewed to Cooley's statement that the apparatus was indeed different, and that he felt DeBakey had not given its development his attention. "If you don't have a man who will go ahead and take the risk," Liotta said, "then my work is valueless."

Reporters also sought out Dr. Charles W. Hall, who had been Liotta's co-director on the DeBakey artificial heart program, but who had left to take a position in San Antonio before the Karp operation. "About one year ago, we started designing on paper a sac type, pneumatically energized pump to be used for total heart replacement," Hall said a few days after the scandal erupted. "Dr. Cooley never worked with us on this project. But DeBakey called us in periodically to make changes or to try to get the research speeded up. Until I left in January, several hundred lab operations had been performed to test various parts of the pump for blood interface and electronic problems.

"During the period from July, 1968, to January, 1969, the artificial heart was used with some success, in four calf operations, the longest of which lived 40-odd hours. But we had never satisfied ourselves that it was ready to be used clinically. . . . Technical errors caused air embolisms. There was always a great destruction of blood cells and improper internal-flow configuration caused stagnation. The heart used in the Karp operation appears to be the same model we worked on."

Was it possible, reporters asked, that Liotta could have designed and built an entirely new model for Cooley? Not likely, said Hall. How could Liotta have done work for Cooley in four months of nights and weekends that it had taken him five years of working for DeBakey full time?

Houston's medical community was sharply divided. One group held that Cooley's use of the artificial heart was a brilliant scientific advancement. The patient in question was dying, and he lived for 65 precious hours with the mechanical pump doing the work of his heart. He regained consciousness, he spoke to his wife, he was alive! Science would not progress unless someone dared to put the mosquito on his arm, they said. A second point of view was that Cooley and Liotta were striking back at years of slights and harassment from DeBakey. A third group considered it an act of betrayal and a severe breach of ethics. There were carefully laid down guidelines to follow in surgery of an experimental nature. Cooley clearly had not followed them. He had made his plans in secret, he had not sought permission from DeBakey, the senior investigator of the artificial heart program, he had not asked for permission to perform the surgery from the Baylor Committee on Research Involving Human Beings, a group of doctors who can theoretically be called into session on 30 minutes' notice to ponder a request, even as a patient is lying on an operating table. "It would not have done any good to call them," said Cooley in private. "Mike dominates the committee and they would have automatically turned me down."

A letter promptly arrived addressed to DeBakey from the National Heart Institute. Written by Dr. Theodore Cooper, director of the Institute, it demanded in curt language a full explanation of the affair:

"The reports in the news media indicate that the artificial heart implanted by Dr. Cooley was developed by Dr. Domingo Liotta. Our grant records indicate that Dr. Liotta's salary and, to a substantial degree, his research, is supported by grant HEW 05435.

"This being the case, I would like to request that the Institute be provided with summary data on the testing and evaluation of this particular device in animals prior to clinical application.

"Also, as you know, current department guidelines require that projects involving human subjects be approved by local committees for human investigation. Was the protocol for the clinical application of this device reviewed by your local committee?"

Investigating committees looking into the controversy proliferated rapidly in the Texas Medical Center. Hearings were held before the Baylor Committee on Research Involving Human Beings, before a hurriedly organized blue-ribbon panel of doctors and scientists who would report to the National Heart Institute, and before an extraordinary commission reporting to the medical school's lay board of trustees. Even Congress rumbled of an investigation as to what was happening with taxpayer money in Houston. DeBakey leveled the indictment in blunt language:

"Application of an unproved device . . . into a human being for primary experimentation before its safety and effectiveness have been proved scientifically in animal experiments is a breach of scientific ethics." The ball was in Cooley's court. Disprove it.

Although the various committee hearings were all conducted in secret—the first time, someone remarked, that anything relating to heart transplants was not filmed with movie cameras—the essential positions of the two sides emerged.

With what one committee member called an "almost patrician manner," Cooley set forth his case. Another told a friend that Cooley seemed "polite at all times, mannered, responsive, in absolute control of himself, supremely confident, even proud of what he had done. . . . He seemed at a loss to understand why he was not being congratulated, rather than investigated."

Cooley said he had become concerned the previous autumn over the increasing scarcity of donor hearts. Leo Boyd had waited eleven weeks for his. Others had died while waiting, still more had gone home untransplanted when their money or patience had run out. Cooley admitted that he knew Liotta was fully committed and in the hire of DeBakey, *and* being paid a salary from the National Heart Institute. But Cooley had proposed at their private meeting that the Argentine surgeon develop something different for him. He wanted a sort of halfway house, an artificial heart to keep a dying patient alive long enough to find a human heart donor. Cooley in his testimony more often referred to a "resuscitative pump" than to an "artificial heart."

"I talked to Dr. Liotta about this idea," said Cooley. "I felt he was as well versed as anyone. I talked to him about the possibility of helping me to develop such a device. Dr. Liotta expressed a willingness to do so."

But why had he not informed the senior investigator, DeBakey, of the arrangement? the committees asked. "Having met with nothing but negative replies to anything of this nature," Cooley said, "and being determined to develop this device, we did not make a formal report." Cooley made several veiled, somewhat sarcastic remarks about his relationship with DeBakey in the Baylor program. At one point he said, "Let me remind you that my position is rather awkward in the surgical research labs. Apparently my abilities more or less have been overlooked in the medical school." After Christiaan Barnard's first transplant, there was, Cooley said, "a great furor here to create a transplant committee at the medical school. . . . I was not invited to be on the committee—but I had no feelings about it one way or another. It gave me a certain independence which I relished."

The artificial heart was tested, Cooley said, by implanting it into seven calves. Though all died, one lived 44 hours. This seemed enough experimentation, he said, "to get this thing on." The use of the apparatus in a human came about only because the man lay dying on the operating table and there was no donor heart available. The artificial heart was there, its large console was there, the patient was there. "Everything came together at once," said Cooley, "*everything*." And, in something of a side-bar remark, Cooley said he had heard that the Russians were planning to use an artificial heart, and he wanted American medicine to be first.

In his most impassioned remarks, Cooley reminded the investigators of his long experience within the human heart, of the thousands upon thousands of judgments he had made. "I have done more heart surgery than anyone else in the world," he told a reporter in a statement that seemed to sum up his case. "Based on this experience, I believe I am qualified to judge what is right and proper for my patients. The permission I receive to do what I do, I receive from my patients. It is not received from a government agency or from one of my seniors."

DeBakey built a careful case against Cooley. Amassing an array of witnesses, documents, invoices, medical sketches, illustrations, diagrams, even careless, forgotten remarks by Cooley that he had made in past speeches—remarks such as his once calling the artificial heart "impractical wishful thinking," and "science fiction"—DeBakey charged:

—That Cooley deliberately lured Domingo Liotta away with visions of a promised land, which must have seemed overwhelming to a man who had spent more than half a decade inside a surgical laboratory.

—That the Karp operation was well planned in advance and not a life-or-death one-minute-to-midnight decision made in the operating room. Indeed, the large console power source is not standard equipment in an operating room, nor are the movie cameras and equipment necessary to photograph an operation from start to finish. One Baylor surgeon said he was asked by Cooley days prior to the operation to participate in it.

—That the seven calves used in the artificial heart experiments all died of severe kidney failure brought on by the device, which should have been a warning that the machine held potential peril for a human. The calf that lived 44 hours was, according to DeBakey, "essentially a cadaver from the time of implantation."

—That Cooley did little but change the valves in the artificial heart to make it different from the one that DeBakey thought was being developed exclusively in his own laboratories.

—That no appeal for a donor heart was made until the day *after* the artificial heart operation, when Karp's wife went on television. What DeBakey left unsaid here was that if Cooley was truly using the mechanical apparatus only as a resuscitative device, he should have made an instant appeal.

—That by using the human heart flown in from Massachusetts to replace the artificial one was the waste of a "scarce organ."

—That DeBakey was shocked and grieved that such an event had taken place within the confines of Baylor.

An observer of the days in which the hearings were held recalled DeBakey as "a man possessed . . . possessed with the need to punish Cooley for what he had done." His eyes, the man said, were "on fire."

Vengeance for DeBakey was quick, and it would have appeared, thorough. Liotta was fired from Baylor, though immediately hired by Cooley for his Texas Heart Institute and empowered to begin a new artificial heart development program. Cooley himself resigned, with sadness, from Baylor, the school he had served for eighteen years. His reason, he said, was that he would not sign the newly imposed restrictions of both the school and the National Institute of Health on experimental human surgery. It was not that he disagreed so much with these guidelines, he said privately, but that he felt if he signed them, he would be bowing to DeBakey. Baylor itself, and its president, were cleared of any inattention and misuse of federal grant money. All the official blame—the guilt—was placed at the neighboring doorstep of Denton Cooley. He was even found guilty by his local medical society on eight counts of "publicity," to which he pleaded speedily, and wearily, "guilty." None of the decisions against him kept him from his surgical practice, and he returned to the operating rooms with renewed vigor, still puzzled about the uproar. There were no outward marks of his flogging, nor had anyone challenged his surgical ability.

But DeBakey would not let the matter drop. Scores of angry letters went out to physicians and hospitals not only in America but in foreign countries, spelling out what Cooley had done and what the investigations had proved. More than one major scientific society felt the wrath of DeBakey when it scheduled an appearance by Cooley (much in demand) to speak on the Karp operation. One such meeting gave Cooley a fervent, standing ovation. DeBakey withdrew many of the classic motion pictures from Baylor's film library of Cooley's famous open-heart surgery in children, some of the definitive work in the field. Suddenly no more reprints were available of papers coauthored by the two men. When *The Harvard Lampoon* published a satire on transplant mania, writing maliciously of a surgeon in Texas named Desmond Coma, who transplanted everything, DeBakey's office photostated copies and mailed them out, thoughtfully underlining the "D" in Desmond and the "C" in Coma, in case anyone missed the point.

His name was not to be spoken, printed, or, it would seem, remembered. Five times Cooley telephoned DeBakey. Five times he left his name with the secretary. "I felt we should at least declare a truce to discuss the future of our respective institutions," said Cooley. "Even the Vietnamese declare a Christmas truce." But DeBakey never called back. "Even when people have a particularly nasty divorce," observed Grady Hallman, "they sit down and divide things up and arrange what's best for the children. But Mike refused to even speak to Denton."

Once, months later, the two men found themselves in the same room at a medical meeting in San Francisco. Everyone present felt the tension might suddenly shatter, that the two men would break from the clusters of admirers who surrounded them, that they might stride toward the center of the room and clasp hands and return to Houston as one, a uniting of their strengths, their skills, their destinies. Cooley, it was said, looked twice across his shoulder at De-Bakey. But the older man, it was further said, no longer acknowledged that Denton Cooley was either present, or even alive.

CHAPTER

15

The transplant year in Houston's two hospitals essentially lasted from May 3, 1968, when Cooley first transplanted Everett Thomas, until April 7, 1969, when he used the artificial heart on Haskell Karp. Both Cooley and DeBakey did another transplant or two after that, but none lived very long and the spirit was gone. "It ended with a whimper, not a bang," said cardiologist Jim Nora.

What did it all prove? It proved that the surgeon was eminently capable of lifting a heart from one man and sewing it into the chest cavity of another. It also proved that the rest of medicine was not yet ready to take it from there. It had been thought that the transplanted heart would behave like the transplanted kidney, that the body would struggle against the foreign organ, but eventually, with the aid of medication, accept it. Immunologists learned that the heart is a peculiar, particular organ, not only a pump, but a creature of some internal, unknown majesty—its depths not fully divined by a hundred-thousand microscopic slides and tissue examinations. Moreover, the heart, unlike the kidney, could not be put back onto a machine to tide it over during a period of rejection.

The transplant year legally defined death, which, curiously, had not been legally defined before, as it related to medicine. In 5,000 years of man's history, a definition had not been required. Legislatures in more than forty states hurriedly passed laws with varying definitions of life's final act. The American Medical Association passed a resolution setting up guidelines for those who would transplant. "The cause of death," resolved the AMA, "must be evident and of an irreversible type. The fact of death must be established and must be demonstrated by adequate current and acceptable scientific evidence in the opinion of the physicians making the determination. The determination of death in organ donors must be made by no less than two physicians not associated with the surgical team performing the transplant." The Texas Legislature concurred with a similar bill to protect, its sponsor said, "not only the patient, but the surgeon."

Transplantation blemished more than one distinguished career. A heart surgeon in Asia was brought up on criminal charges that he deliberately neglected a dying patient so that he could take the heart and use it in someone else. Another surgeon in America was sued for $1 million on similar charges of neglect.*

On the third anniversary of human heart transplants, December, 3, 1970, the American Heart Association totaled up the worldwide statistics and announced that 166 heart transplants had been done since Barnard opened the door and that only 23 were still alive, giving the procedure an overall mortality rate of more than 85 percent. Ten of the 23 still living, however, had survived for more than two years. The only place in America where there remained enthusiasm for the procedure was Stanford University. Dr. Norman Shumway could count nine transplants alive out of the 26 he had performed. In the fall of 1970, he superseded Denton Cooley as the surgeon who had done more heart transplants than any man in the world.

Shumway could not resist criticizing Cooley in a published interview. Shumway said: "It's not a surgical business, primarily. If it were merely a surgical exercise, they'd all have survived. In trans-

---

* *In April, 1971, Mrs. Shirley Karp, widow of Haskell Karp, sued Cooley, Liotta and St. Luke's Hospital for damages totalling more than $4 million. Although Mrs. Karp signed a release for her husband's surgery and afterwards publicly praised Cooley, she claimed in her suit that she did not understand what she was signing and that her husband was "the unfortunate victim of human experimentation." She further claimed that neither she nor her husband knew that the artificial heart had never been used in a human being.*

plants, you see diseases come into being that people had never dealt with. You need a lot of people with a lot of disciplines. You can't have Sonny Jurgensen [the professsional football quarterback] win games without a good line in front of him. You can't do transplants in a specialty hospital. The leader of the team can't be a character who dominates every conversation and never has anybody around him who can't contribute beyond him. Bright people must be heard. The guy that does cultures in the lab must feel as important as the guy who sews the heart in. . . . Cooley said, 'The prescription for success in heart transplants is "cut well, tie well, get well."' . . . That's naïveté. The problems come after surgery. They're not surgical problems."

Shumway had been the man whom American medicine thought would usher in the era of transplanted hearts. Instead he became the principal surgeon to survive it. Mercifully, the race was no longer a race. The spectators had gone home; all the runners save one had dropped out. He could afford to take all the time he needed to reach the finish line.

In Houston, Jim Nora and the other Baylor scientists interested in immunology and rejection went back to work. Using tiny, tweezerlike instruments and a miniature scalpel, Nora and his team began removing the hearts from pure-bred white mice and transplanting them into the ears of other mice. There they usually thrived and could actually be seen on the face of the ear, beating away under a thin layer of membrane. The purpose was to test various formulas of immunosuppressive drug administration and the mouse's tolerance of a foreign body. One mouse, a favorite of the scientists, lived for several months with another's heart beating in his ear.

With no great enthusiasm, Nora discussed with me three potential breakthroughs in managing transplant recipients against rejection.

The first, he said, would be to cook up a pool of transplanation antigen that could be made from pieces of the heart, thymus, and spleen taken from cadavers, plus pieces of thymus taken from a living patient during open-heart surgery. Hopefully, all possible human antigens would be dwelling within these bits and pieces and could be made into a serum. In what is called "low zone" induction of tolerance, the patient about to receive a donor heart would receive over a period of weeks carefully planned injections of this serum, beginning with infinitesimal amounts, working up to larger and larger doses—in much the same way an allergist desensitizes a patient to ragweed. Theoretically, a recipient could accept any new heart, even a badly matched heart, because his body would already have all known antigens swimming about and would not recognize the new heart as "non-self," but "self."

A second and corollary procedure would be to create the same serum from a pig's organs, inject it over a period of weeks into a human patient, and then transplant a pig's heart into the man.

A third, crash plan or "high zone," method would be to go ahead and transplant a heart into a dying man, then inject him with a serum made from the cadaver donor's liver, spleen, and those pieces of the heart not used in the operation. "The patient would be so flooded with soluble antigen that his body would be unable to recognize and reject the new heart," said Nora.

When would the immunologists be ready to go ahead with one or more of these procedures?

"In point of fact, about five years," he said. "In point of medical and moral priority, 50." When the transplant era ended in his hospital, Nora was so burdened with guilt and disenchantment that he made plans to move himself and his family to Haiti, where he and his wife, a hematologist, would work for a year at the Schweitzer Hospital. An unexpected second child appeared, however, and Nora instead stayed in Houston and began writing an angry novel of transplantation set in a Southwestern city and called *The Upstart Spring*. "It was a purge for me," he said. "Nothing else." In December, 1970, he would accept a position as head of the pediatric cardiology department at the University of Colorado and move to Denver.

"Was the transplant year a major disappointment of your life?" I asked Cooley one quiet summer morning in 1970. He was sitting in his second office, a small, windowless room in the basement of St. Luke's; behind him was a color portrait of the transplant team made the moment after an operation, with an inscription from Gide, "Man cannot discover new oceans unless he has the courage to lose sight of the shore." Cooley is the kind of man who will answer impertinent if not cruel questions, and he did not hesitate. He explained the failure by believing that it was not a failure. Our conversation:

"There are many blind alleys we must go down in making progress," he began. "If you're charting unexplored territory, you can't expect to be riding down a freeway. You've got to go out there where there are no paths, many times you may go through one canyon and meet a cliff. To get from Plymouth Rock to San Francisco Bay, the pioneers didn't go straight over the hill to the valley on the other side. Sometimes blind alleys may be only temporarily blind, subsequently we'll blast them open."

"Then I take it you have no regret over the transplant year?"

"No." Emphatic. "I don't think I have any regrets about having tried. I followed to the best of my ability those principles of selection of patients, of taking desperately ill patients whose hearts were in advanced deterioration. I can't recall any of that group that I could do anything more for today. So that's reassuring to me."

"None of them would be candidates for the coronary artery bypass surgery which seems so popular these days?"

"Out of the twenty-one, I can't think of any. Because they had ventricular aneurysms, diffuse areas of scar tissue that would make them entirely unsuitable for the bypass. We didn't stretch the indications for transplant surgery. Even though some of the patients may have had their lives shortened by a few months, none of them had their lives shortened by a matter of years. The few months of life would have been unsatisfactory. . . . I look back on transplants as just one of those procedures which we tried, and for the time being, discarded."

"Was there a time when they all began coming in and rejecting and dying when you felt your skills had deserted you?"

"Well, I couldn't help but ponder why some other surgeons have had patients who are still alive, after two years, and my longest survivor was sixteen months. But I think that our initial results are as good as anyone's. What happens to them three months later is not a reflection of the surgical technique! Surgeons don't control these things anyway. . . . People say, well *his* results were worse than others, but look at some of the things we tried. We tried a newborn infant, nobody else had pulled one off the table. We got a heart *and* a lung out of that one. We did a five-year-old. We took people who were flat-out dead and put a new heart in, and they lived! It was an opportunity, a time for testing things, and, by God, we tested them."

Would Cooley consider using the artificial heart again?

"Of course! I'd have implanted it two weeks ago if I had had one ready to go. There was a man with a healthy body who died on me because his heart was diseased. It wasn't time for him to die. I'll tell you one thing—by the end of this decade we won't be letting people die on our tables. Some patients will live for a year with an artificial heart inside them."

Only in a laboratory one floor above DeBakey's surgical suites was there unqualified enthusiasm in Houston for transplants, not because they were a valuable surgical procedure, but because—as an ironic side product—they provided a tantalizing clue to the very nature of heart disease. The principal investigator there was a bio-chemist named Arnold Schwartz, a friendly, engaging scientist, one of the hundreds drawn from the eastern United States, lured by the aura of DeBakey. "I enjoy being a pearl on DeBakey's necklace, but it is a symbiotic relationship," he said. "DeBakey never comes around because he knows who is producing and who isn't."

Schwartz long ago had accommodated himself to the lesser role of working as a researcher in a house of surgery, even though he was and is often skeptical of the surgeon. "Surgery to me is not creativity," he explained. "It's plumbing, very exquisite plumbing, but plumbing. What we do with the hearts *is* creative. When you start humanizing something in science, I'm not sure you can create."

During the time of heart transplants, Schwartz—for the first time in his career—was able to obtain fresh heart tissue for study. "Short of going out and killing somebody and taking their heart, I had never been able to examine fresh tissue. When DeBakey and Cooley started doing transplants, I went right into the operating room with a mask and gown on and they snipped off a little piece for me. They called me 'The Ghoul from the School.'" Schwartz also was given the en-tire recipient heart to study after the natural owner received a new one.

His continuing study since 1962 was called "Ion Transport in

Cardiac Muscle," in which Schwartz had concerned himself with the chemical process that makes the heart contract and expand and push blood throughout the body. With fresh heart tissue, he was able to process all the membrane systems in cells which have anything to do with ion transport. Ions are electrolytes—calcium, sodium, potassium —and when a heart beats, it is the reflection of these ions moving in and out of millions of heart cells. After studying 25 recipient hearts that were diseased, Schwartz made a surprising discovery.

"Every heart has a calcium binding system that must contract and relax over and over again for 70 or 80 years," he explained. "In the 25 defective recipient hearts we studied, *in every single one of them,* this system was defective. This was learned only since heart transplants began.

"Now we are studying the hearts of dogs and rabbits and we are discovering the same defective system, which you could call a chemical imbalance. This is a breakthrough—this could be the cause of heart attacks. Diet and stress and all the rest could aggravate a condition, but the main cause of a man dropping dead from a defective heart might be a chemical imbalance within his electrolytes."

If Schwartz becomes convinced that his discovery is of the magnitude he is beginning to suspect it is, then he and the Baylor pharmacologists can explore possible drugs or hormones to prevent the calcium binding system from becoming defective. His work would seem to be the most hopeful thing salvaged from the transplant year.

Between Methodist and St. Luke's hospitals in Houston there is a cluttered, cut-up area of little more than a hundred yards across, which some of the younger doctors refer to as "No-Man's Land." In the summer of 1970, bulldozers and heavy machinery needed for construction work going on at St. Luke's roamed the small area. Trucks with girders, cement mixers backed in and out, sometimes throwing a shower of gravel against a small tin shack called Animal House, so named because experiments with animals are sometimes conducted there. Often workers in hardhats leaned against the shack to smoke or look at blueprints. It was a place of such ordinary anonymity that I passed it, parked my car within a few feet of it a hundred times and never noted its sand-colored presence.

But within Animal House is a narrow closet, two feet or so wide, and if one had a key to the closet, one could open it and find seven ordinary shelves, crowded with white plastic containers, the kind women use to store food in large freezers. Within these containers are the 22 transplanted hearts that were given to 21 people (Everett Thomas got two) who came to St. Luke's Hospital for the operation that ignited men's dreams that December night in Cape Town. The hearts are a grayish yellow now, rubbery from the alcohols and formaldehydes preserving them. Someday there will be a Museum of the Heart in Cooley's fine Texas Heart Institute and perhaps these will be displayed for the student and historian.

Each of the hearts showed in autopsy the same signs of rejection, signs unique to transplantation: hemorrhage along the lining of the heart, thickening of the heart walls, mottled appearance of the myocardium. Each of the hearts was studied, probed, analyzed, pushed under microscopes, wondered over, despaired of, and finally put into the white plastic containers and taken to a locked closet in Animal House, where they were stored, and where, for weeks at a time, no one even thought of them.

If you stood very long in front of the closet and looked at the shelves, you would gaze first with curiosity and then with wonder and then with sadness, and after a while your eyes would sting from the fumes of the acids. I saw the hearts and I felt a strange unsettling and I walked hurriedly away from the ghosts and into the blazing Texas sun, feeling my own heart pounding in me.

PART THREE

CHAPTER
16

My sons flew from New York to Houston as summer began in 1970 and I met them at the airport. Both were pale from the long Eastern winter and shaggy in the land of short haircuts. We drove to my apartment near the Medical Center; chattering, proud father and progeny, of baseball statistics and unpleasant instructors who had assigned summer homework and all things important to boys nine and twelve. Both had received physical examinations by an eminent woman pediatrician in New York to fulfill requirements for admission to summer camp in Texas and once again a doctor had heard the unknown in Scott's heart. Their mother had told the pediatrician that Scott's murmur would be heard by the sophisticated ears of the Houston heart world and the doctor seemed elated. "Be sure and have them send me a report, and an x-ray, or if. . . ." She left the rest unspoken. Not even *she* would speak of surgery.

At my apartment, the boys stripped off their flannels and blazers and striped ties in seconds and leaped yelling into the pool. Their happiness, plus the fact that Houston's largest park and zoo lay unex-

plored directly across the street, seemed reasons enough to delay talk
of the stethoscope for a few days at least.

Cooley and Liotta were to be decorated by the Spanish government and Monday surgery was concluded by 2 P.M. so they could
change into formal dark suits and somber ties for the ceremony in the
auditorium of Texas Children's Hospital. Cooley had arranged a
liaison with the Spanish medical community in which he would receive around $3 million for his Texas Heart Institute and in return
would train Spanish cardiologists and surgeons in Houston. It was
said that research money was so scarce in the United States that
Cooley had to go to a foreign source to find some. There was further
talk in Houston that some of Cooley's contributors had grown disenchanted after the artificial heart controversy. Cooley discounted
this and blamed the slowness of his fund-raising to the general business recession of 1969–70.

Cooley would also perform guest surgeries in Madrid and Liotta
would spend considerable time there developing a new artificial
heart and testing it on Spanish calves, which were a great deal
cheaper than those in Texas. Cooley and Liotta were to be awarded
the Grand Cross of Alfonso X, who had ruled Spain from 1221 to
1284. The decorations were in honor of "meritorious service to medicine," for their use of the artificial heart in Haskell Karp fourteen
months before. If the prophet was without honor in certain parts
of his own city, then at least a foreign government recognized the
achievement.

On the afternoon of the award ceremony, the Texas Children's
Hospital auditorium was filled with nurses, doctors, patrons of the
hospital, and the many children of the two honorees. There was a
decided "hooray for our side" feeling in the room. From Madrid had
come a dashing representative, Dr. Cristobal Martinez-Bordieu, who
was also the Marquis de Villaverde, in addition to being the son-in-
law of Francisco Franco. Struggling in English, the Marquis made
a brief speech explaining that Alphonso X was known as "a monarch
of the highest intellect" and that the award named after him had
originated in 1903, given at first to those who achieved excellence in
the literary field and later changed to science. Only four Grand

Crosses of Alphonso had been awarded since 1944 and the new members of the order, Cooley and Liotta, were honorary knights and entitled to be called "Excellency." Franco himself had authorized the decoration of the two Houston doctors, the Marquis said with flourish.

"The implantation of the artificial heart was a moment in history," said the Marquis, and with that pronouncement he draped a crimson sash from the neck of each man, embraced him, and pinned on a striking red and white medal. The next day, the nurses called Cooley "Sir Denton" and "Your Excellency" in the operating rooms.

The great annual kiddie rush had begun. Open-heart surgery is, in the majority of cases, an elective procedure. Many parents traditionally waited until the summer and school vacations to bring their children to Cooley's table. On one Monday in early June, Cooley scheduled correction of three Tetralogy of Fallots, the classic "blue babies." Each had received a preoperative "briefing" from a nurse named Diane whose job was to explain to the child facing open-heart surgery what would happen to him and what he would look like afterward in the Recovery Room.

"On Monday, Dr. Cooley is going to fix your heart up," said Diane to a solemn-looking boy of eight named Kenny from Mississippi. She sat on his bed and talked to him directly. "On Sunday night they'll give you a Phisohex bath to make you very clean, and then before you go to sleep you'll have shots—one to kill germs, one to make you sleepy. You won't remember anything until you wake up *after* the operation, and then you'll look like this."

Diane pulled from her shopping bag a Raggedy Ann doll with carrot-colored hair and tubes and wires sticking from her, a doll that seemed to have broken apart many times and, out of love, been wired back together again.

"The first thing you'll notice is this mouthpiece. There'll be a funny machine beside your bed and it's to help you breathe. This machine breathes for you while you're getting your heart fixed up and they'll keep it going until you get all waked up in the Recovery Room. You probably won't like the mouthpiece and you'll bite down on it. But it's important that you not be afraid of it and not fight it. The best thing to do is take a few big deep breaths through the tube and go back to sleep. Okay?"

"Okay," echoed Kenny, his eyes as large as half-dollars. He glanced anxiously at his mother, who nodded reassuringly.

"The nurse will come by your bed and ask you to squeeze her hand. When you can do that big and strong, then she'll take the tube out of your mouth. . . . Now, have you seen an oxygen tent before?"

"Yes, ma'am."

"They'll probably put you inside one. It'll be like a glass playhouse, it'll be cool. There may be some mist inside to help you clear your chest so you can cough good. This is important. If they ask you to cough, you'll promise to do your best and cough for the nurse?"

"Yes, ma'am."

"Your stitches," said the nurse, pointing to the doll's sewn-up chest, "will look like a zipper, or a railroad track. And you'll be hooked up to a little TV set so we can watch your heart rate. Maybe you can lean your head around and see it, too. There'll be another tube here"—she pointed to the doll's arm—"or maybe here"—pointing to the foot—"to feed you and give you medicine."

The nurse gave Kenny the doll to hold and ponder over for a few moments. He gave it quickly back to her; it was an offending object. "Do you have any questions, Kenny?"

"Will I have shots?" Children fear shots more than the surgery itself.

"Only those on Sunday night. After that they'll give you all your medicine through an IV tube like this."

Kenny smiled for the first time.

"One more thing. The first day after your operation, you'll be real sleepy. You'll get to see Mommy and Daddy that same night. Then you'll be moved over to another Recovery Room on the same floor with only children around you. Maybe you can talk to them and there's a window you can look out. Probably in a day or two you can come back to this room. The most important thing, remember, is not to fight the breathing tube and to cough when they ask you, and turn when the nurses tell you to. And when you come back to this room, promise me you'll exercise your body. It's like when you get hurt playing ball or something, it doesn't do much good to stay home in bed. You've got to make your heart work again."

Diane shook Kenny's hand and hurried from the room. She had another appointment down the hall and she was worried because a Korean child had flown in from Seoul for surgery and there was no Korean interpreter immediately available to translate the briefing with the doll.

On Sunday night before the three Tetralogy of Fallot cases were scheduled, an emergency case appeared at St. Luke's and John Zaorski squeezed him into the crowded schedule. The patient was an Italian clerk from Rome, a thin, once handsome man in his forties who worked for the police department. His name was Nino Bergoni, and his wife, Maria, half-carried him into the hospital, her handkerchief wet and dirty from his vomit, her own face weary from tears and hysteria. Neither spoke a word of English but somehow it was learned that the trip had been arranged through the office of Pope Paul, that they had gotten lost during a seven-hour layover at Kennedy Airport in New York, and that Nino almost had died on the flight to Houston. Zaorski slapped him instantly into Recovery, where nurses could keep an around-the-clock vigil and try to keep him alive long enough for Cooley to operate in the morning.

The three Tetralogy of Fallots, including Kenny, were done by noon without complications and each was sent to Recovery with a newly plumbed heart by the surgeon who had refined the hellish operation to where it was routine. Nino would be done after lunch and I went down to pediatric cardiology, where the technicians were already complaining, mildly, about the flood of youngsters pouring into the hospital.

There Jim Nora was catheterizing a poignant case, a four-and-a-half-year-old boy, son of a Midwestern psychologist and his wife, who, in addition to having the gravest congenital heart defect—the AV commune—was suspected of an equally rare genetic disorder, which caused mental retardation. The only sound the child could make was a high-pitched wail, the cry of a frightened kitten. The medical name for it is *crie de chat*, "cry of a cat," named by a Frenchman who first encountered it.

It took Nora more than an hour just to get the catheter into a vein. "This is the end of the line for so many kids," he said. "They've been worked up and studied and cathed elsewhere so many times that they just have no veins left when they get down here. All I'm finding is scar tissue."

Nora paused and looked at the child, struggling beneath him. "He's a nice little boy, but the parents refuse to accept any diagnosis of retardation," he said. His face was enveloped by sadness. "He makes a sound which the mother insists sounds like 'mama.' She says he is only slow to develop." Now there was the weary edge of frustration to Nora's voice, which, as he went on, became understandable. Nora would have to spend several hours of his and his staff's time, as would Cooley, attempting to repair an almost impossibly damaged heart— and even if the procedure was successful, the child would live but a short, fitful life, bringing pain and cruelty to all concerned. And he would probably never speak, other than to make that chilling noise of a cat crying. "Other places wouldn't touch this kid," said Nora. "They'd consider it a waste of hospital resources. At the University of Wisconsin, where I used to be, they could do only four open-heart operations a week. But here Denton does forty, and he's good enough to try anything. And if the parents want it, he'll attempt it." (Ironically, this child survived surgery, a procedure that has an 80 percent mortality rate. But another child with the same AV commune disease who was completely normal otherwise died a few weeks later on the operating table.) The pediatric cardiologists frequently study mentally retarded children with heart defects, in particular, Mongoloids. Nora willingly recommends heart surgery for these, even though their anticipated life span is also short and discouraging. "A Mongoloid child often becomes a sweet, loving member of a family. Operating on a congenitally damaged Mongoloid heart seems somehow worth the effort," he said.

I had missed earlier that day one of the most unnerving and delicate procedures in the heart world, one that Nora and the other pediatric cardiologists do in the catheterization lab, not the operating room. When a baby is born with transposition of the great vessels of the heart—the same defect that Cooley had repaired in Pamela Kroger in April—it may be necessary to operate immediately and create a hole between the chambers of the heart. The surgeon is creating a new, and less serious defect to enable the blood to circulate better. Theoretically, the child will live until he reaches the age of four or five and is better able to withstand open-heart surgery and having his blood circulated through the pump-oxygenator. "The trouble was," explained Nora, "a lot of kids didn't even survive that first operation and died within a few weeks." A cardiologist named Rashkind at the University of Pennsylvania developed a technique in which a catheter is stuck into a baby's arm and threaded gently up the arm and down into the heart. At the end of the catheter is a tough plastic balloon, which, when in exactly the right position, is blown up. The cardiologist then takes a deep breath and yanks on it forcibly, ripping a hole in the heart. Though fraught with tension, the procedure seems to work surprisingly well; better, in fact, than surgery. "But it still scares the hell out of us when we yank," said Nora.

Nino Bergoni's operation began at mid-afternoon and Cooley was in an expansive mood, perhaps because the three Fallots had gone so perfectly that morning, perhaps because he had raised at long last enough money to award the contracts on the eight new operating rooms for the Texas Heart Institute.

As he put two valves into Nino's heart, deciding against a third because triple-valve replacements have had discouraging results, Cooley talked of the news that Dr. Walton Lillehei, pioneer of American open-heart surgery and chairman of Cornell's department of surgery at the New York Hospital, was resigning. Lillehei also had been criticized for his heart-transplant program. "I remember one Christmas Eve a year or two ago when the phone rang," said Cooley, pausing a moment to peer at the new mitral valve he had sewn into Nino, "It was old Walt calling. He says to me, 'Denton, I'm fixing to do a heart-lung transplant. You did one. You got any advice?' 'Yeah,' I say. 'What is it?' 'Don't.' "

When Nino was taken off the pump, his heart began to fibrillate. "We've got a circus movement," Cooley said, his voice becoming serious. Gwen, the supervising nurse, was at his side instantly with the electric paddles and with one jolt, the heart regained its normal rhythm. Another nurse came into the operating room and said that Nino's wife, Maria, was giving everybody a hard time. All afternoon the hospital staff had been chasing her out of the surgical area, but at that moment she was standing outside the "Do Not Enter" doors with her nose pressed against one glass, and holding up to the adjoining pane her wallet, which contained photographs of Dr. Cooley and Pope Paul, side by side.

"I met the Pope once," said Cooley. He was satisfied now that the heart was beating naturally and as he began sewing up the pericardial sac, he recounted his conversation in the Vatican study.

"The Pope said he had followed our work and had kept track with all the transplants and he endorsed our work with but one exception. 'What was that?' I wanted to know. He said he was concerned about the definition of the donor's death.

"Do I infer, your Holiness, that you do not accept brain death? 'I would prefer,' he said, 'that the heart also be stopped.'

"That would be putting the rights of the dead over the rights of the living, your Holiness."

At 7 P.M., the parents of the three Tetralogy of Fallots were permitted in to see their children and despite the shock of the tubes and wires and monitors, none fainted. Maria, however, came into Recovery just as Nino was starting to awaken from the anesthesia, his body quivering and in spasms. She assumed her husband was in terminal throes, that she was witnessing his death rattles, and she began to moan and tear at her rosary. Just then a well-meaning priest ambled by on his nightly rounds, glaced at Nino's chart, saw that he was Catholic, and idly made the sign of the cross. Screaming, Maria collapsed and had to be helped from the room, with two nurses and a frustrated resident trying to find the Italian word for "normal."

Within 48 hours, Nino was recovered sufficiently and had gained enough strength to be transferred to the sixth-floor Intensive Care Unit. In celebration, Maria positively blossomed. From the haggard, sobbing woman in a dowdy, farm-wife's dress, she appeared in a stylish green and white jersey ensemble with a gold belt and gold shoes. Her face was beaming as she waited outside the Intensive Care Unit for the six daily visits she was permitted to make to her husband's bedside.

Late one afternoon that mid-June week, I was leaving the hospital to collect my children from a friend's pool when Grady Hallman stopped me. Hallman was a perfect partner and alter ego for Cooley.

Quiet, confident, slim, youthful, the surgeon took the spotlight only when he conducted and played trombone solos for the Heartbeats. On those occasions, Cooley was in the back row playing string bass. In the hospital, Hallman worked almost privately in Operating Room 3, doing the aneurysms and vessel work and less glamorous operations, while Cooley drew the acclaim down the hall. I had sought several times to speak with Hallman at length, but he had always seemed too busy.

"There's a patient of mine you might want to see," he said. "It's a case of a man with a lethal lesion who got here in time." Hallman introduced me to an elderly, strong-looking man from Arkansas named Allgood, who had thick white hair and whose room was filled with flowers, candy, and get-well cards from back home. Allgood sat up in bed and shook hands all around. "I'd get up and do a little dance, but I just got back from walking around the halls," he said. A few days earlier he had been in bed in his Arkansas home when he felt a "terrific pulsating in my lower abdomen." The local doctor suspected an aneurysm but advised that he could wait for surgical attention until after a grandson's high-school graduation. "But the back pain got so bad that they told me to get to Houston as fast as possible."

Allgood had arrived on a stretcher in the back of a chartered Lear jet and Hallman operated immediately. It was, he saw, the kind of rupturing aneurysm that had killed Albert Einstein. Death would have come within hours, or minutes. "The Lord just wasn't ready for me to get gone from here," he said. "I am a strong believer in Jesus Christ and the Baptist church. A real Christian goes to the limits of his ability and then the Lord takes over. With help from Dr. Hallman."

Hallman had slipped out of the room during the story and when I found him he was at the nursing station writing medication. It was past 9 P.M. and he was still making rounds. "That's a rewarding case," I said, gesturing toward Allgood's room. "He's a nice old fellow," Hallman said without looking up from a chart, "I'm glad he got here when he did." Since Hallman had himself broken the ice, so to speak, I asked if we could have a lengthy conversation one evening soon. The young surgeon thought about it and finally nodded. He gave me a tentative date a few nights hence.

It was my hope that I would learn not only something about Hall-man and his work, but that he would illuminate the mystery of Cooley for me. After months of false intimacy about and around the man, of standing in his surgery and witnessing every detail of his art, his speech, his silences, his rounds, his almost reluctant entrances and exits from patients' rooms, I knew little more of him than did those who entrusted their hearts to him.

When Hallman and I finally sat down and had that evening's talk—not a few nights but a few weeks later, just before Hallman went away on vacation—I knew little more of Denton Cooley. But the conversation itself cast a light on the craft and business of surgery. It was the most candid, and in some ways most frightening, five hours I had spent in Houston.

We had drinks and dinner in a new private club, one of the hundreds scattered throughout Houston, a city where the state law said that mixed alcoholic drinks could not be served in public places. When I had gone to college and worked as a newspaperman in Texas, it was a brown-paper-bag society. One dined in the finest restaurants with a wrinkled bag on the table concealing a bottle of whisky. It was within the law to bring the bottle to the restaurant and use it as a centerpiece. The restaurant would even furnish a glass, ice, and mix. But in more recent years, private clubs with instantly acquired memberships had prospered under the archaic, Baptist-enforced law. Houston wanted so desperately to become a big-time city—and in so many ways it is—that authorities tolerated the illegal imbibing.

I had become accustomed to Houston's heart doctors giving me courteous thirty-minute interviews during office hours and beyond that the impression that I was stealing highly valuable time. Now I had one after hours.

"How long do you have?" I began with Hallman. It was 7 P.M.

"As long as you need."

Hallman had gone to the University of Texas and then to Baylor, where, in the early 1950s, he became enchanted by internal medicine. The surgeon had not yet come into his prime in Houston. "The men I met doing internal work were intelligent, they spoke well, they seemed to be investigators. I was convinced my career would be among them. But when I was a senior I was assigned to the charity clinics and there I sat all afternoon . . . interviewing women with boring chronic illnesses . . . problems that needed weeks or months of tests to learn the answer, if there was an answer. Problems that could perhaps *never* be solved. When I rotated onto the surgical service, I was instantly struck by the positive action, by the possibility of spotting a problem and doing something immediately!"

One of the top five graduates in his class, Hallman chose an internship at Wesley Memorial Hospital, in Chicago, and for a time switched his interest to anesthesiology. "I saw myself as both an administrator of drugs and a great teacher and writer." But once again surgery lured him back. It was not his participation in surgical cases. For an intern, there is scant stimulation in working up patients, writing histories, finding x-rays, holding retractors, or maybe cutting a stitch now and then in the operating room. It was the invitation from a great chest surgeon for Hallman to spend an afternoon seeing patients and making diagnoses in the surgeon's Chicago office. "I didn't even have anything to wear," remembered Hallman. "I asked the surgeon what I'd need, and he said, 'Just wear what you've got.' So I put on a zip jacket and spent a fantastic afternoon. When it was over that night the surgeon and I compared notes; our diagnoses generally matched. He was seriously interested in me. He was everything I had wanted to be in medicine. That one afternoon turned me onto surgery for good."

Hallman thereupon wrote DeBakey "a flowery letter, telling him how much I admired the accomplishments of the Baylor Department of Surgery." DeBakey was now a prominent surgeon, world-known among doctors, but without the glamour that would soon come. Hallman was promptly accepted and spent seven years in residency: four in general surgery, three in chest.

"What kind of cases does a first-year resident do?" I asked. I had been spending my days in Houston among those at the top of the profession and had no idea what the beginning man went through.

"Well, you fix hernias, take out appendixes, remove hemorrhoids. You do procedures commensurate with your level of talent, with a senior man supervising you all the time. You do work that the patient thinks the senior man is doing.

"In the second year, you graduate to gall bladders, you explore gunshot wounds, do amputations, thyroidectomies. Third year you should be up to gastrectomies, radical breasts, colon resection. And by the fourth year, if you make it that far, you're administratively the head of the service. You get the pick of the operations. You can take out entire stomachs, do all the vascular surgery, pneumectomies, etc."

During his three-year chest residency under DeBakey, Hallman went through the traumas indigenous to the work. "My third child was born in another hospital during this time and had it not occurred on a Sunday morning, I wouldn't have been able to slip away from DeBakey long enough to see him. I didn't see the kid again for another three months. My car was stolen when I was on the unbroken 90-day shift and I couldn't even get out to see about it. I lived on sandwiches, fried pies, and Fritos. I got a vitamin deficiency and my tongue turned fire red. I figured that what I went through was the supreme test of human endurance. But there came the day that it was all over. I made it through."

"Did DeBakey shake hands and show his appreciation?"

Hallman looked startled. "He's not that type. He never tells anybody thank you, or good job. He's never done that in his life."

Toward the end of his chest residency, in July, 1962, Hallman analyzed carefully the problem of where he would go to work.

"I never even considered trying it on my own because I knew if I hung out a shingle, the only cases I'd get would be from relatives. So I said to myself, 'Of everything you've done and seen in medicine, what is the most interesting, most challenging, and potentially the most financially rewarding?' I answered myself, 'Denton Cooley.' I got up my courage and went over and cornered him and blurted out, 'You don't have any help. I want to go with you. DeBakey's always had a right-hand man, or several.'" Everyone knew that Cooley had always been a loner.

Cooley's reaction, Hallman remembered, was looking as if he were in an enormous hurry to get on with what he had been doing before the young surgeon had trapped him. But Hallman pressed. "You say to yourself, 'What can this unknown doctor offer me?' Well, he can do surgery that's sent to him by people who know him, he can do the clinic cases, and he can co-write a textbook on pediatric heart surgery and make you first author. . . .'" With that, Hallman remembered, "Denton's eyes lit up." A book was needed in the field, Hallman said hurriedly, and where could a better one emerge than from Cooley's case histories and data?

Thinking he had interested the great heart surgeon, Hallman went away to await an offer. Days, weeks, months passed and not a word was sent from Cooley. One afternoon, in despair, Hallman saw Cooley backing out of the hospital parking lot and flagged him down. "I made the pitch again, but he didn't seem too interested. He was running only one operating room then and doing about three or four cases a day. Maybe, I see now, he didn't want the competition."

As a distinctively second choice, Hallman applied to DeBakey and it seemed he would be hired as a junior man when "a strange thing happened." The *Houston Chronicle* wanted to interview a surgical resident for a feature story on medicine. Someone recommended Hallman as the subject and a woman reporter interviewed him. "She wrote mainly about the financial problems—she wanted to know how many suits I had, and I said one, a $25 number I picked up in a bargain basement. She wrote that my shoes were resoled, that we fed a family of five on $5 a week, that we had a $25 car, that we had a hand-me-down television set sitting on a packing crate. . . . A surgeon I knew told me, after reading the article, 'You couldn't buy that kind of article for $1 million. It makes you out to be the all-time champion underpaid, starving, dedicated young doctor.'"

Not two days later, Cooley telephoned and asked if Hallman still wanted to join him.

"What did you do for him at first surgically?" I asked.

Hallman made a circle with his index finger and his thumb. "Zilch," he said. "He gave me nothing. Surgeons always feel they can do everything best and that they have no need for anybody else. Sort of by accident I started doing arteriograms when Denton didn't have time to do them. I did three or four a day, at $50 each, and for the first time in my life, I started making money at medicine. And I did my very rare private surgical case. Mainly I spent the next five or six years researching that book and when it was finished—and successful—I suddenly had offers from Mayo to New York. There was a lot of fertile ground in 1967. I was all set to take one of them when Denton announced he wanted me to become his partner. He had got a second operating room by then and his case load was exploding. Now I think I made the best decision. Financially, it has become the most attractive place in medicine. And it's gratifying that people come from all over the world to be operated on by us. . . . I'm able, in fact, to operate as much as I want, which very few surgeons can say. And our band, the Heartbeats, is a tremendous emotional outlet for me."

Hallman fell silent for a minute and when he next spoke, he revealed himself. "The only thing I'm not is the complete boss . . . my own man. . . ." DeBakey had looked over his shoulder once and had seen Cooley and if Cooley were to look over his, there would be Hallman. My attention was caught and held by what Hallman said in the late hours of the evening. It began with my observation that patients agreed so quickly, almost mutely, to surgery, that Cooley was in and out of their rooms *and* in and out of their hearts.

Hallman smiled. "Denton believes in the blitzkrieg approach. He storms into a patient's room, tells the guy he needs the operation, and he thinks the problem can be fixed, and the patient is so overwhelmed by this that he agrees."

I had once seen a patient decline surgery and Cooley had seemed disappointed; yet he had made no attempt to change the decision. He only nodded and walked brusquely from the room. "There's no hard sell," Hallman said. "First of all, we don't need the business. We're not going to miss the case and the schedule will be filled anyway. Secondly, most of the selling has already been done. By the time a patient sees us, he's already been to at least two or three other doctors. Thus the phrase which I'm sure you've heard over and over again, 'That's what I came for . . . the sooner, the better.' If a guy doesn't want surgery, then it's his decision. Denton doesn't try to change anybody's mind."

But why the volume? Why the relentless pursuit of first place? Was there not a peril in the sophisticated, impersonal, medical assembly line?

"He who rides a tiger can never get off," answered the young surgeon. "It's intimately tied in with pride and arrogance, as well. When a referring doctor sends us a patient and we're too busy or too exhausted, what are we going to do? Send him over to DeBakey? Refer him to Mayo? To Ochsner? If we don't do the surgery, who is? A patient pays us an enormous compliment by wanting to partake of what we offer—and we do it better than anybody else. *We play the violin concerto better than anybody else down here because we've played it more times.* We do so many cases that our patients get well! The same case might go to Boston or New York or Mayo and get sick, have clots, lose legs, or die. We have *perfected* heart surgery."

But, I wondered, how then does the artist avoid destroying himself physically if not emotionally by playing so many concertos?

"Denton has a need, a compulsion to work. Nobody in the world works harder than he does. There are few people on earth who have unlimited capacities for work. He's one. . . . I'm another. Besides, surgery *is* like show business. We're performing in there. No matter how exhausted one becomes, you get up the moment you enter the operating room. It's like a second cup of coffee, a pep pill, a dexedrine, an amphetamine. . . . You see the patient lying there before you and a second wind comes to you. When we were doing transplants, we often worked all day and all night and all the next day. The sheer drama of the situation was a stimulant."

What of the shield between Cooley and his world?

"Anybody who has the exigencies of Denton doesn't have the minutes left to get close to anybody. Nor do I. I used to love to read . . . it was my supreme joy, and now I have no time to read." Hallman's voice was, for a moment, sad. He seemed to be speaking not to me but to himself. "A person who has no time to read has no time to come close to anybody or thing. When you commit yourself to becoming a heart surgeon, you must divorce all human relationships— wife, family, patients. . . ."

My face must have reacted and asked a silent question. Hallman must have anticipated it, because he was ready with an answer.

"Any physician who lets himself become emotionally involved with the patients disables himself. This applies more particularly to the surgeon. In OB-GYN there are rarely deaths . . . in dermatology, no deaths. . . . The GP has an occasional death but they're usually old, worn-out people who are ready to die anyway. The only weapon we have against death is the ability to convince ourselves that we've done the best possible surgery.

"People must die! It's no good to speculate that somebody else might have done a better job, that somebody else might have cut this or that differently. . . . But unless *you* do the surgery, how then are you going to become good?"

I interrupted. "Then what you're saying is that patients must be. . . ."

Now Hallman cut in. "Sacrificed."

He said the word softly.

I fumbled. I was, in truth, stunned. "I was going to suggest an easier word," I said, "like 'pioneers.'"

"Sacrificed is a better word. Some patients must be sacrificed to the God of Experience. Excellence comes out of experience and nothing else. A doctor can reach the supreme pinnacle of technique, but only after he has done many, many cases and perhaps participated in many, many deaths. If every patient in the world got the best possible surgery, then there would be no resident program and, consequently, no new surgeons. Some surgery simply must be done by those who are less than perfectly qualified."

I looked down, away, not for a waiter, not to watch the people in the club going about the business of drinking and talking and living, but to hide. I wanted no more truth. Hallman pulled me back. He was not done. He needed to get it all out. "It's true!" he said. He waited until I nodded. Of course it was true. But truth is not necessarily a defense.

"A surgeon who is the best," he went on, "is a surgeon who has gained the most experience." He reached into his memory and found a part he had long since shut away. "And some of the first few people that surgeon operated on are dead. This is blunt talk, but every surgeon would say the same thing. . . . I know a lot of people who are dead today because I operated on them early in my career. If I could do them tomorrow, they'd be alive. . . ."

We talked for another restless hour. I don't remember what we talked about.

I was a father with a son whose heart made an alarming sound and I was a man with access to the great heart surgeons of the world. There were so many judges to stand the boy in front of. I weighed them all in my mind—the exasperating, ruthless genius of DeBakey, the cold beauty of Cooley, the energy, the strength of tested youth that was Diethrich, the chilling honesty of Hallman. Bricker slept beside his patients. But only Nora had wept. I had seen him try to understand why children are defective and die, I had seen him unable to control the pain of having to deliver the ultimate message. I had heard his sorrow of the transplant year. I was not a liberal seeking comfort in another liberal, nor did I equate tears with ability. But tears as I knew them in Houston were strength, tears could mean compassion. I wanted a doctor to lean on. Nora, the pediatric cardiologist, was not even a surgeon—but in the land of kings, I asked a commoner for his favor.

I made the boys dress up and sent them back to comb their hair. Permission had been obtained from Mrs. Sylvester, the operating room supervisor, for them to stand in the gallery and watch Cooley operate. That was the lure. I had expected them to watch with interest for a few moments and then be repelled by the wound. But they stood entranced for half an hour asking questions about anatomy and mechanics and movement, which, after my months in the chambers, I could answer. "Is that his heart?" Scott asked, pointing to the throbbing object encircled by the hands of Cooley and his men. I nodded. "How much will he hurt?" the child asked. Not a great deal, I hoped. I looked at my watch. It was time.

"Come on, Scott, as long as we're here, I'd like for this doctor to listen to your heart." I was pulling him from the gallery. He didn't want to leave.

"Not again," the little boy said fretfully. His heart had been heard in Paris and an EKG had been taken. The machine with its wires and attachments had frightened him, but there had been no pain. "*Très curieux*," the cardiologist had murmured.

"He's just going to *listen*. I promise."

"Can I come back and watch Dr. Cooley some more?"

"Yes. If the nurses will let us. It depends on the case."

"Can't we do it another time?" He was stalling.

"No." Firmly. Parental. "We're here. Let's get it over with. It's all arranged. It'll only take a minute. He's a very nice doctor."

We walked down the stairs. Scott was squeezing my hand. It was a game we had always played. He would grip me as hard as he could and I would feign at last that he was hurting me. "If I'm going to be a surgeon," he said, relaxing his pressure, "I'll have to start taking care of my hands."

"I thought you were going to be a baseball player for the Mets."

"But I've changed my mind. I want to operate on people."

Nora was holding clinic. There were parents and their children stacked up outside his office. A baby was yelling in her mother's arms. There was a strangeness, a cast to the infant's face that alarmed her parents. Nora would run a genetics test to see if the baby had mongolism. They had learned of the possibility and their expressions showed that their jeopardy was perhaps graver than mine.

He worked us in ahead of the others. He accepted the tough handshake from my son and winced as if he knew how to play the game. He was good with children. He knelt down and looked the boy directly in the eye. It impressed me that he did not bend over. "Can you take your shirt and tie off for me, Scott?" My son looked at me with suspicion. It *was* going to take more than a minute.

Nora placed the stethoscope on the smooth, unblemished young chest and listened. "Okay," he said, with no commitment. Neither yes nor no. What was he hearing? My thoughts flew to the boy's mother. Her sister had been born with a heart defect, which Cooley had repaired in his first years of open-heart surgery. Surely *her* side of the family had passed down the abnormal seed, if there was to be one. I needed someone to blame.

Nora moved the stethoscope up and down and instructed Scott to hold his breath. I heard the baby crying outside. I was annoyed. There must be silence for the doctor to hear. Slowly he took the instrument away and let it drop to his chest; it hung there against his white coat and a thousand years crept by before he raised his head and spoke.

"It's Still's murmur. A *false* murmur. It is a vibration of the pulmonary valve. Here, listen for yourself."

Nora handed me the stethoscope and placed its disk against Scott's heart. The beat was firm, but in its aftermath, a quick hiss, a spurt of steam from a radiator.

"Put your shirt on, Scott. It's all finished." Nora seemed happy to gently slap the naked back of a whole child. I gave Scott a quarter and he went with his brother Kirk to find the Coke machine.

"There's nothing to worry about. The vibration will be gone away by the time he's thirteen or fourteen."

"Then there's no need to even think about surgery . . . ever?"

Nora shook his head.

"But what about those other doctors? He's been listened to in New York and Paris. . . ."

"Don't blame them. We get a lot of business out of Still's murmur. The state of the art is such that they just don't recognize some of the things we've heard a thousand times."

Nora walked me out. "I assure you it's nothing."

"Nothing?"

Nora was smiling. His face lit up the room and all of my world.

Scott watched surgery for the rest of the morning. He was fascinated, entranced as I had never seen him, by the grace and strangeness of Cooley's operating room. "Dr. Cooley works very hard," he said.

"He works all the time. Being a surgeon is more than you think."

"What did my heart sound like, Dad?"

"Like a bass drum." I put my hand to my chest. *"Boom! Boom! Boom!"*

My son laughed; we left the hospital and went swimming. Scott stood on my shoulders and dived into the water, he prowled the bottom and attacked my legs, he pestered his brother, he squandered every moment of the day because he was rich, blessedly rich with time, newly endowed by the heart doctors.

CHAPTER
17

Bergoni, the Italian police clerk, watched his wife brew espresso in a tiny pot she had found in a hardware shop near the hospital. She had pronounced Houston hospital coffee to be not only inferior in taste but potentially damaging to her husband's liver. "It might give him a setback," she announced to one of the staff who spoke Italian. All day long she prepared the thick, heavy coffee of Italy, poured it into thimble cups, dumped in three spoons of sugar, and gaily served it to the doctors and nurses who attended her Nino. She was annoyed they would not let Nino sip a bit of *vino blanco*.

Few operative results had so delighted the hospital. Maria was radiant, as strength was rushing into Nino's wasted body. He seemed an old man when he had been carried vomiting into St. Luke's ten days before. Now his eyes sparkled and there was color pushing away the grayness. The only thing that worried the staff was Maria's unhidden rekindling of romantic desire. There was a day bed in the room and Maria was permitted to sleep nights on it, but one of the residents had to caution her, tactfully, about invading *Nino's* bed for the immediate future. "It's been two years since they had a married life," said the doctor. "She's probably forgotten what it's like."

Early in July, a reporter from Johannesburg, on an American tour to write about transplants and heart surgery, interviewed Cooley.

"June was the busiest month in our history," Cooley said. "We did 115 open-heart operations, our all-time record."

On another day, another reporter wanted to know why Norman Shumway at Stanford was continuing to do heart transplants, in light of the generally discouraging world results.

"Maybe he doesn't believe in coronary surgery," was Cooley's reply.

The surgical fellows were all talking of how enthusiastic the chief had become over the grueling coronary-artery bypass operation. Only last April, they insisted, Cooley had thoroughly disliked it. Now Cooley was saying things like, "This operation is second only to sexual intercourse." On some days there were as many as four scheduled on the green blackboard.

"He's committed to it now," said Dennis Cokkinos, the Greek cardiologist. "And once he's committed to something, watch out. He'll bomb all those other guys and their statistics."

Cooley had done seven in three days and the seven men in their forties and fifties all seemed to be making excellent recoveries. "People are saying that you have become enamored of this operation," I ventured, "that you'll soon be doing more than anybody else in the world."

He laughed. "Well, there's a possibility, I guess, that I will. It's true that others have identified with this procedure before we have. We did, however, an ancestor to this operation in 1964, some of the initial work on kids who had congenital anomalies. Lately we haven't been considered very bold and aggressive with coronary surgery. It took a while before we were able to impress ourselves with the efficacy of the procedure. I think this is important. I won't take someone else's word for it, because the same individuals who are promoting this operation have promoted others in the past which proved to be relatively worthless."

A few days later he expanded on the subject in a speech given to about forty doctors from Texas and Louisiana:

"I believe there is no other area of surgery that has enjoyed more fads than coronary surgery. In the past twenty years there have been operations which had largely psychological effects and which were very lucrative to the surgeons who did them. This led to the charge of charlatanism.

"This new operation, the coronary bypass, is the most tedious, most meticulous operation known to the surgeon. We must sew in a field no bigger than two millimeters across, sometimes only one. I believe we must have a quiet bloodless field. Therefore I clamp the aorta.

"This operation seems to bring relief. It is not a psychological effect, but a *true* physiological effect."

But it would take the judgment of years before the surgeon could win all cardiologists over to his point of view. One, a prominent internist who practiced in downtown Houston and who had little to do with the heart hospitals of the Texas Medical Center, could barely conceal his fury. "I've had patients who simply do not need surgery, who defy my will, and who go directly to these 'great' heart surgeons. They suggest my diagnosis is based on jealousy. We're not allowed our opinions anymore!" He was speaking to a visitor and his voice must have thundered through the closed door into the outer office and waiting room.

"With each new procedure, each new one supposedly better than the last, the surgeon rushes in and cries that it is the greatest, the newest, the most hopeful procedure, and he *decries* the one before it. We've seen this so often, we've been burned so often that we've become dubious of the surgeons waving the flag and beating the drum.

"But imagine the potential here! Every man in America over the age of 45 has some coronary artery narrowing, but many of them are asymptomatic, that is, they have no pain and can function normally and productively. I'll tell you one thing, we'd better watch the surgeons because sooner or later they're going to suggest that everybody, and I mean everybody, must have this spectacular operation to *prevent* having a heart attack. They're going to recommend that everybody have an arteriogram as part of the annual checkup, and an occlusion will show up on an arteriogram, and *WHAM!* Onto the table."

The cardiologist was out of breath and lit a cigarette. He insisted that he did not inhale. "We think surgeons lie like hell about their statistics," he said. "The best results usually come from those who want to get their names in the papers. They're even touting something new called an infarctectomy in which they take a near dead man immediately after his heart attack—the fellow is in shock—and rush him into the OR and cut out the dead part of his heart and bring the other parts together and stitch it up. The patient survives the operation, sure, but he dies twelve hours later in Recovery of 'cardiac arrest.' That's crap! The patient dies, that's all! Use of the term 'cardiac arrest' is actually a camouflage to cover the fact that the patient died from what the surgeon did to him."

Two interesting and poignant pediatric cases arrived at Texas Children's within days of one another. First came a three-month-old baby in a coma brought in by his mother. While the pediatric cardiologists began drawing blood and ordering all manner of tests, someone suspected an overdose of something and asked the lady if she had given the child any medicine. She had indeed—twelve aspirins that very morning. The baby had a bad cold and she decided to storm it. She had great faith in the value of aspirins and regularly lined her brood up each morning and gave them one aspirin each. "Well, your baby's dead," said one of the pediatricians, who was so upset by the woman's stupidity that he could barely speak to her. It was the third death from acute aspirin poisoning that the hospital had seen in three months.

Next arrived Eric, a frisky black baby of eighteen months who got into his own trouble. Born with a ventricular septal defect in his heart, he was being watched until he grew large enough for open-heart surgery. He was also taking one digitalis tablet a day to slow down his fast heart and strengthen it. One morning he climbed up on his mother's dressing table, discovered the bottle of digitalis tablets among her cosmetics, and chewed up sixteen—more than half a month's dosage. The overdose slowed down his heart to the point where it was barely beating when the mother finally brought him in, empty bottle in hand. While one doctor put the comatose little boy on dilantin to stabilize his membranes (the same drug used in epilepsy,) potassium, and intravenous fluids to step up his urination, another went outside to the waiting room and scolded the mother. Later he was talking of the case and said that massive dosages of digitalis used to be a classic—and perfect—way of committing murder. "The victim's heart would stop, it would appear to be a heart attack, and there was no way to measure digitalis in the blood stream. But the lab boys have discovered new methods to foil Agatha Christie."

The danger was that Eric would go into heart block or arrhythmias. After a few days of intense observation, his heart picked up from a dangerous low rate of 60 to 100 and he was pronounced out of danger. Upstairs he delighted all the floor nurses by popping balloons in his bed and by making furious faces at everyone who passed by his door. There was one good side effect. His liver, which had been oversized from the bad heart, shrank from all the digitalis, and his lungs cleared up.

I followed but two more patients through Cooley's surgery and each became pieces fitted to the puzzle he remained to me. But once they fell into place, the picture was incomplete.

One was a 47-year-old college dean, the other a six-year-old girl. They came from separate cities to enter the hospital within hours of one another and they had their operations a day or two apart. I grew to respect the courage and wisdom of the man, I fell irrevocably in love with the beauty and good nature of the child. I followed one down the mountain and watched death, I ran with the second up the other side to the summit and claimed life. I think I even saw Cooley break toward the end when he paused, then hurried past the room of the one who was dying. But it was but a dropped, perhaps forgotten, moment.

Nobody on Cooley's staff was glad to see Clement Fisher return, not because he was an unpleasant man—he was, in fact, a cheerful and tolerant patient—but because he appeared at St. Luke's in late summer needing a *fourth* replacement of the same mitral valve. The other three that Cooley had sewn into his heart over the space of nine months had, for one reason or another, grown defective. That he required his fourth open-heart operation in such a short period of time was discouraging to all concerned.

Fisher, a college dean, was a tall, spare man with china blue eyes and a wide East Texas drawl. He told the investigating doctors that his heart trouble had begun when he was thirteen and running track. "The coach felt the longer and harder we ran," he said, "the more wind we'd have for the dashes. One day I felt something pull inside my chest." The Houston cardiologists were more inclined to suspect childhood rheumatic fever than a rare traumatic injury to the heart, but Fisher insisted that as far as he knew he had never had the disease. "My mother took me to a doctor a few months after that day on the track, and he said I had strained my heart and that I should spend the rest of my life in bed. I did no such thing. Believe me, I've had a great life! But I always paid extra insurance premiums for a heart murmur."

In 1940 when he obtained a marriage license and had a physical examination, the doctor diagnosed a "leaky valve." "He said it was flapping in there like an old barn door," Fisher said. "At that time the only thing a fellow could do was accept it and live with it. Nobody was cutting into hearts then. To tell the truth I never paid much attention to the damn thing until a couple of years ago when I was helping the workmen move some billiard tables in the student union building and I strained so much I went into my office and lay down. I went to see my doctor who chewed me up and down. 'You durn fool, you've done it again,' he says to me. 'I oughta kill you, but I'll write Denton Cooley.'"

Fisher flew to Houston in the autumn of 1969, where the cardiologists discovered that the valve was leaking so much blood that the heart was functioning at about 30 percent of capacity. Cooley replaced the defective natural valve with a plastic and metal one and sent Fisher home as he had done with hundreds of successful patients before. "I hardly got off the plane before the new one started leaking," Fisher said. "My arteries and veins stuck out like cords of steel on my arms and legs because the heart was throwing so much pressure on them. My heart had been functioning at that 30 percent capacity so long that when Cooley fixed the valve and sent the heart back up to normal, the valve just couldn't stand the pressure and tore loose."

In December, Cooley tried a fascia lata valve, one made from the tough tissue of the patient's own inner thigh.

It seemed to be holding well until Fisher was released from the hospital and drove to the Houston airport. There he was told that his scheduled flight had been cancelled but if he hurried to a gate at a far-off end of the terminal he could catch another airplane. Fisher picked up his own suitcase and that of a friend and ran down a long, polished corridor. "By the time I stepped off the plane at home," he said ruefully, "the second valve had torn loose."

Three months later, when his body was strong enough to accept a third major operation, Cooley sewed in another valve, but the tissue around the valve was becoming so necrotic that it did not hold. Now Cooley was faced with the unpleasant job of trying to make a fourth one stick. "I don't think anybody's ever tried four before," said John Zaorski. "I've never seen it in the literature."

Fisher remained good-natured, unlike some who return to hospitals for a re-do, convinced they were victims of inept medicine. (A few years before, my appendix burst during lunch one afternoon in New York and I was operated on that evening by a well-known and expensive surgeon. In the three months that followed the wound would not heal and I had to return for a second operation to scoop out the silk stitches—which I was "spitting," they told me—and infection. I was, with no challengers, the supreme grouch of my floor.)

Before his second valve replacement, while being examined by Cooley, Fisher presented the surgeon with a small bottle of glue to make it stick. Cooley had laughed and said he would use it intravenously. Before the third, Fisher asked Cooley what kind of warranty the apparatus carried. And now, as he waited the fourth, Fisher sent his wife out for a zipper.

Tammi, who was only six, had enormous deep-set blue-gray eyes. Her body was tiny from a deformed heart, but she carried it with grace. One moment she would be sitting on her bed playing a card game called "Hate," the next strolling down the hall watching the other heart kids play. But Tammi would only watch. She held herself aloof and if she was frightened, some check within her held it from sight.

Cooley leaned over her and listened to her heart. He nodded noncommitally and smiled at the beautiful precocious little girl and her parents, a barber and his wife.

Outside he told the entourage of young doctors that Tammi had a bad AV commune, the highest-risk heart surgery. Earlier that summer, Cooley had won one of them—the boy who cried like a cat—and lost one. Few surgeons in the world would bother, or dare, to try. "Most places would send her home to die," said Dr. Ugo Tessler, an Italian resident who was new to Cooley's service. (On July 1, most of the foreign doctors had left and a new dozen had come to take their place.)

Tessler walked on, frowning. "She won't last through surgery."

"How long can she live without it?" I asked.

"She won't. She's going to die." Tessler's voice was flat and final.

Cooley was on his way down a flight of stairs, on his way to see Fisher, but Tammi was on his mind.

"I'd like to think that no patient is too sick for surgery," he said almost to himself. "I'd also like to think that the only ones we turn away here are the ones who don't need surgery."

"Will you attempt the operation on Tammi?"

"We'll see."

Trying to make Fisher's fourth valve stay in place, Cooley used a technique of overlapping heart tissue around the mouth of the valve and sewing it doubly tight. He went out after the operation and told Mrs. Fisher, a stylish, attractive woman in a Chanel-type suit, that he felt sure it would hold.

"I've heard that before," she said as he walked away. "I've heard everything before." She was weary and her eyes were red from lack of sleep. She had not, in fact, slept well for nine months of failing valves.

During Fisher's operation, Tammi was taken for the third heart catheterization of her young life. Five months after she was born, a hometown pediatrician detected a murmur. "I've heard these before," he said. "I can only give you an educated guess, but I don't think there's anything to worry about." But when she was one year old, Tammi fell short of breath, refused to lie down, to stop crying. Her mouth and lips turned blue; cold sweat popped out on her forehead. She was in classic heart failure. Her mother drove the baby in panic to the hospital, where she was slapped into an oxygen tent and put on digitalis to strengthen the tiny heart. When she was three, Tammi was brought to Texas Children's Hospital in Houston for her first catheterization, which revealed the suspected AV commune. And in the June of her sixth year, the Houston cardiologists catheterized her again. Jim Nora had told Tammi's mother, "We've gone as far as we can without doing something. . . . She doesn't have much time left."

During the next two months the barber and his wife addressed themselves to a cruel dilemma: whether to keep the merry, prankish child at home and seize the time left and crowd it with love—or return her to a hospital where there was the darkest pessimism. "We lived with it for a long time," the mother said while she waited in the snack bar with a cold cup of coffee, waiting for Tammi to be brought back from the catheterization lab. "Dr. Nora had told us the last time that we needn't fear anything sudden happening. She wouldn't go . . . overnight. But now I know the gradual decline is setting in. I can see her slipping every day. If Dr. Cooley feels there is a chance, only a tiny chance, then we'll put ourselves in his hands and the Lord's."

The night before, after Cooley had dropped by to listen to her heart, I had returned and visited with Tammi. There seemed no sickness about her other than her thinness; she fairly burst with life and humor. "Dr. Cooley's going to fix your heart up," her father said, as we played Battle with her well-worn deck of cards.

"Mmmmmmmm," said Tammi, showing me how she could shuffle, "I think I may wait. When I'm about nine, I *may* let him." She was a princess dispensing favor. She dealt out a hand quickly and began sorting her fate. She looked up and affected a pensive look. "But I *would* like to beat John in a race," she said, explaining that John was a very fast child who lived in her neighborhood.

We walked down the hall and stopped to look at a bulletin board outside the nursing station, which was filled with photographs and letters from children who had happily returned home after heart surgery. Tammi's eyes found and lingered on a picture of a solemn boy with a large incision of his chest. The stitches had not yet been removed.

"Would you look at that," she said. "They cut that little boy all up."

On the third postoperative day, Fisher threw a small clot to his brain which, hopefully, only temporarily paralyzed his side. He also developed jaundice and turned a dull yellow. His eyes seemed on fire.

Zaorski listened to his heart and shook his head with weariness. I asked what was happening but he said he had to hurry to another case.

Dr. Chuck Mullins, one of the many able pediatric cardiologists, did Tammi's catheterization with Nora coming into the room now and then. "This kid's heart seems so malformed that the catheter just flops from side to side," he said. He was gently moving the catheter at an incision in her arm and watching its passage into the heart over a television screen. The wire moved murkily into the shadow that was the heart. "Her heart is a mess," he said. "It's outgrown her body." The shadow was enormous. It was evil.

Nora had stopped for a cup of coffee just outside the catheterization lab. I asked him what causes congenital defects in children. "There are many reasons," he answered, "largely unknown ones. The major one is probably the hereditary predisposition. Then there are environmental triggers—bacteria, radiation, insecticides in food, maybe the mother took too many drugs like dexedrine during her pregnancy to keep from getting fat. Women take such incredible things during pregnancies. We're highly interested in viruses now; we're studying blood from newborns to see if the baby had an infection in the womb."

"What about when the mother gets German measles?" I asked.

"That's the most widely known cause, when a mother has German measles in the first trimester of pregnancy. But it accounts for the smallest percentage of defective hearts, less than 5 percent. If a woman does have German measles during the first ninety days of pregnancy, there is a 60 percent chance the baby will be born with congenital heart disease."

When the catheterization was over and before Tammi was sent back to her room, Dr. Mullins talked with her mother. He tried to conceal his despair. "There's really no choice," he said. "Either you take her home and wait—or you consider surgery, even though the risk is high. Very high. She simply has no heart reserve left. The heart can't rally on demand and produce more output. You and I can run, climb stairs, rally to fight an infection. But her heart can't. A cold might be a catastrophe. And I don't know a way in the world to keep a child of six away from infection."

The mother seemed confused. "But are you recommending surgery?"

"Dr. Cooley will have to decide and then it will be up to you and your husband. I just wanted you to know what I think."

Later that afternoon, the fellows in the coffee room were talking of Tammi and Don Bricker heard the conversation.

"She's going to die," he said. "I wouldn't touch her."

"Then what would you do?" someone asked.

He threw up his hands in surrender. "Give her to Denton."

The buck stopped at the surgeon's desk in his tiny cubbyhole overlooking the operating room. The collected wisdom of fifty centuries of medicine was at his finger tips—Tammi's x-rays, the films of her catheterization, the sheets with the chemical equations, the recommendations, the calculated guesses. But only the man who held the knife could decide whether to bring the child to the operating table that he could see from his desk.

He went to her room as she was eating and asked her parents to follow him into the corridor.

"I think I can help her," he said. No one had really expected him to turn the child down.

"Would you do it if she was your little girl?" The mother asked.

"If she were mine, I wouldn't want to. But I'd do it." I had heard him give the same answer many times, almost automatically. But on this hot summer night the voice lacked its positiveness.

Both parents nodded as one.

When the surgeon went away, Tammi piped up, "Dr. Cooley didn't say anything to me. I must be too beautiful."

That night during dinner at his home, John Zaorski talked of Fisher. "I think I heard a leak today," he said. "I'd guess the valve's torn loose." He added that he was not 100 percent certain. But happily, Fisher's jaundice had cleared up and he was later transferred to a private room. With the yellow cast gone from his body, he was psychologically better and the paralysis from the stroke seemed to be easing. His wife and married daughter were guardedly optimistic.

On the morning of Tammi's operation, Dr. Mullins passed by surgery. He had wanted to watch the procedure, but he had to catheterize the second of identical six-year-old twin blond girls whose Tetralogy of Fallot had been repaired a year ago. Both twins were spectacular successes and were back only for checkups. "I'm crossing my fingers with Tammi," he said, ". . . and saying a few prayers as well. Her heart's as big as yours or mine."

What worried Mullins most was the deteriorating mitral valve, one of the many defects that he suspected in her heart. "Denton can probably sew up the holes, but the valve is the problem," he said. "The surgeon has a completely different thinking on valves than we do. Denton talks about them lasting ten years, but they can also last only five years or five months. The average seems to be about four or five years. I wouldn't want to face a life of having my chest opened and the surgeon into my heart every four years. . . . Because once that valve goes out—it's out. And life depends forever thereafter upon the strength of a piece of metal and plastic."

Tammi watched Diane, the nurse with the Raggedy Ann doll, explain how she would look after surgery and her face grew unusually solemn. At six could a child really understand that which was going to happen to her?

Sedated with Nembutal and Demerol, Tammi was rolled to surgery at 9:30 A.M. She waited briefly for her turn in Room 2. I leaned over the stretcher. I was masked but she recognized my voice. "I'll see you in a little while," I said. "I'll keep the cards warm." She bounced her head up and down. "You may have to deal," she said. "I'm so sleepy." On the table, she struggled against the black mask that came toward her, sending the vapors of cyclopropane and halothane into her lungs. Quickly she was out. Quickly she was still and silent.

She lay nude on the table while the team performed its preparatory ballet about her. The heart within the tiny body was leaping. "Her head almost vibrates every time the heart beats," said one of the doctors. "Poor kid."

Dr. Phil Allmendinger came into the room. A burly, surgical resident from Connecticut, he was spending six months of his third year of residency in Houston beside Cooley. He had arrived on July 1, the change-over date, and in but a few weeks had become overwhelmed by the variety and volume of heart work. "It's everything I had hoped it would be," he wrote to a friend in Connecticut. "Already I've seen lesions it would take a year to encounter back there." Allmendinger quickly won the nurses with his decisions in the Recovery Room; the women made immediate and generally accurate evaluations of the new doctors. "Did you come early to get a good seat?" he whispered through his mask. Already the room was crowded. An AV commune would sell out any operating room.

One of the nurses said that Cooley was in a snappish mood. "I saw it the moment he scrubbed in," she said. Allmendinger knew why. The day before Cooley had lost a difficult aortic aneurysm patient. Also, during the repair of a ventricular septal defect on a two-and-one-half-year-old girl from South America, one of the new foreign fellows had, for reasons unknown, taken the clamp off one of the tubes connecting the patient to the pump-oxygenator. Allmendinger, assisting, glanced down and saw a huge air bubble swimming toward the patient. He made a diving grab for the tube to shut off the bubble's course and put the clamp back on. Cooley saw only the dive and was angry. "Christ, Doctor, everything we do in this operating room has a definite purpose," he said. "Don't you know an air bubble like that would go directly to this patient's brain?"

When Cooley lowered his head and returned his gaze to the field, Allmendinger glanced discreetly toward the fellow who had made the blunder. But the guilty man did not speak up and accept the blame. Rather than squeal on a junior colleague, Allmendinger let it ride. Cooley worked for the rest of the operation in stormy silence.

One of the ward nurses had not helped his disposition on the morning of Tammi's operation by charging in and complaining that six patients on her floor had been told they could go home but that no one had written the discharge medication and papers. "Nurses stab you in the back this way," said Allmendinger. "They should complain to you, but they go direct to the chief." Cooley got on the loudspeaker and acidly told Zaorski, "There are patients stacked up on Three South. Let's get 'em out of here." The general gloom that surrounded Tammi's chances was heavy in the room, and there was a thoracic aneurysm that had to be done after the child. And Hallman was on vacation.

John Russell sliced into Tammi and began peeling back the layers of skin and tissue. The nurse Gwen was hovering behind him preparing the electric saw. "Ready for the saw, Dr. Russell?"

"Just about."

Gwen waited a moment or two. "Ready now?"

Russell nodded. She handed him the saw and he applied its blade to the child's chest. "Okay. Hit it."

The nurse switched on the current and the blade chewed through the breast bone.

"Through?" asked Gwen.

"Yeah." Russell gazed at the heart.

"I didn't hear you go through."

"It's very soft bone. You don't hear the pop in kids."

A visiting doctor standing on a stool shook his head. "Jesus Christ, look at that greedy heart."

Wordlessly, Cooley entered the room. Three doctors stepped back from the table to permit him entry. Hurriedly he put the child on the pump. When her blood was flowing through the tube into the oxygenating machine and back again into her body, when the gross heart was still enough for him to enter, he cut it open, peeled back a flap and stitched it tightly to the thoracic cavity to keep it out of the way. His fingers found the atrial septal defect—one of the suspected holes in the heart—and he began trimming a piece of Dacron to cover it. "The hairy part," Allmendinger whispered to me, giving me a play by play, as he could see better than I, "is the valves . . . whether he'll be able to resuspend them . . . or replace them."

But when Cooley was finished sewing in the patch, his slender fingers moved again inside the heart. He stopped. He re-entered. He stopped again. It was not his custom to stop. His surgery was always a fluid motion. Fifty eyes raced from his face to his hidden hands and back again. What horror had he encountered? Suddenly he smiled. "We have an ostium primum, I believe, gentlemen," he said. There was *not* the second suspected hole in the heart. Nor would the valves have to be replaced. There was only one complicated hole in the heart, an atrial septal defect known as ostium primum. As a sudden storm breaking the August heat, the tension in the room shattered. Some of the visiting doctors even left, as people walk out of a disappointing play. Cooley satisfied himself one more time that the valves were not damaged, then closed the pericardial sac. "This just goes to show that one peek is worth two finesses," he said as he sewed. He was elated. He was, in fact, triumphant. "The cardiologists have been finessing this child all of her life, seeing shadows and pronouncing her doomed and predicting her death. All the surgeon had to do was go in and look. Now she should be fine!"

By mid-afternoon, Tammi was groggily awake and asking for a hairbrush. She returned to her room the next day and 36 hours after the operation was walking about her room. Her recovery astonished her mother. "Mama came in and found me walking around the room and almost had a heart attack," Tammi said, accepting my kiss. "Now let's play cards." Her doll was beside her on the bed; she had had an operation as well, her chest was covered with a large bandage, and tubes dangled from her arm.

The jaundice had come back and Fisher had turned the color of an old coin. It was difficult to talk with him, but he wanted to talk. His voice was raspy. He spoke of the things cluttering his mind—his love of flying, his work at the university, his family, his ordeal. I complimented him on his courage. He closed his eyes tightly and when he opened them there were tears in the yellowness of them. "I've given up many a time," he said. "Nobody knows it. I've laid back and said, 'I quit.' I feared the Intensive Care Unit. I've always had a fear of choking to death—it happened that I almost drowned once—and when they put me in that room full of sick people and stuck the tubes down my throat, I knew they were going to let me lie there and strangle to death. The roof of my mouth is still sore from where I pushed on the breathing tube."

He fell silent for a time. I took it as my signal to leave. "I'm ashamed of what I just told you," he said. "A man shouldn't give up that way. . . ."

The women of his family had gathered. Over the weekend, the men had come, too—brothers, brothers-in-law, sons-in-law. But they had gone away. "Men can't sit in the hospital and wait the way we can," said one of the women. Mrs. Fisher refused to let them move her husband back to the Intensive Care Unit. "He's had enough," she said. She sat outside his room in a chair, leaning against the corridor wall. Before she would go in to relieve her daughter, she would go to the ladies' room and put on fresh makeup and achieve a difficult, but workable smile.

Fisher's heart had slowed down and was betraying his body. Fluids were collecting everywhere. Diuretics were administered to speed up expulsion of the liquids, but they always came back. Tourniquets were tied on his arms and legs to stop the fluids from going to his heart and drowning him—that long hidden fear. But it was an exercise in palliation. Even he must have known.

The last time I made rounds with Denton Cooley he began at the summit. He inspected Tammi's rapidly healing incision and swooped her up for her mother's camera. She challenged him to play cards with her sometime and he laughingly accepted. He seemed almost reluctant to leave her. Phil Allmendinger had already noticed, in the brief time he had been with the surgeon, how much Cooley favored the pediatric cases. "I think he only comes alive when he's with the congenital heart kiddies," Allmendinger said. "They trust him, they don't ask questions, they have rapid healing powers, and they get well quickly. It's usually permanent with them. They don't give the surgeon that tiny, nagging doubt in the back of his head that so often haunts him with the grownups."

As Cooley strode toward the adult floor, he gestured with his head back toward Tammi's room. "That case shows how *necessary* it is for the surgeon to go ahead sometimes when everybody else is predicting disaster. Tammi is fine, there's no more murmur, she's looking good, she's *alive!*"

He walked on and spoke to John Russell. "It makes all the weeping and wailing of relatives worthwhile," he said. "When we first started doing this work, kids died on the table every week. We practically had to wade through hysterical relatives."

He was in fine fettle for half an hour, a pleasant half-hour with a series of bright, sunny rooms and, within, patients and families whose faces were cheered when the surgeon entered. But finally there was the woman sitting in the chair outside a room, and the entourage stopped. Russell looked at the name on the door and said, unnecessarily, "It's Mr. Fisher."

There was nothing to do. There was nothing left for the surgeon except to wrestle with his soul for that last moment. He had already seen his failure, and nothing—neither his hands nor his sorrow—could alter the destination. Mrs. Fisher did not look up. His face sagged and he shook his beautiful head. "Poor bastard," he said softly as he moved on. There was nothing to do but move on to the next patient.

Fisher died the next day.

Tammi went home and five months later, at Christmas, wrote me a letter in New York. "Dear Tom," it read, "I am a Brownie. I marched in the Christmas parade. I did not get tired. I love you. Happy Christmas! Love! Tammi."

CHAPTER

18

Duson Vlaco left Belgrade in the late summer of 1970 and flew a third of the way around the world to Houston for a routine examination of his physical condition and of the heart that two years before had been taken from a 36-year-old man and implanted within him. The heart was no longer a foreign object. Duson's system had manufactured billions of new cells and they had lived and died and had been reborn on the surface of the heart until the organ belonged solely to him. After a fortnight of tests—EKGS, x-rays, blood counts, bicycle pedaling, cardiograms—Duson stopped Ted Diethrich in the hospital corridor and said shyly: "I'd like to get out of the hospital for a day and go swimming at your house."

On the following Sunday, Diethrich held a regular sports day at his home and from noon on, a dozen young surgeons and medical students spent the early hours of the afternoon bashing each other in frontenis, football, water basketball, water volleyball, and bouncing on the trampoline. Shortly after 3 P.M., Duson appeared, accompanied by his Yugoslavian cardiologist, Dr. Anicic. My first reaction to the strange child with the new heart was to recoil and shudder with

pity. He walked happily across the patio on match-stick legs supporting a barrel-like torso. The skinny arms and hands seemed not so
much a part of him but instead hastily attached, like branches slapped
onto a snowman by a child. His head was huge, swollen to a pumpkin
shape by the daily tablet of cortisone still taken to guard against
rejection. There was a buffalo-like hump at the back of his neck, a
thin, fine layer of hair across his shoulders, and purple stretch marks
on his abdomen. Another purple blotch covered one side of his face
and neck. But he shook hands firmly with everyone on the patio and
sat down in a deck chair and smiled with a warmth that washed away
much of the grotesqueness. "I like the Texas sun," he said, tilting the
pumpkin head toward the heat and opening his shirt. Ted brought
him a soft drink and Duson drank it hurriedly. He saw the bicycle of
one of Diethrich's children and asked if he could ride it. Diethrich did
not hesitate. "Have a go at it," he said, and the boy with the borrowed
heart ran to it and climbed on it and rode out the driveway onto a
quiet lane with huge oaks. There were oil-company executives mow-
ing their yards on sit-down machines and women pruning roses and
children shrieking at their Sunday games, but none looked up as Duson
rode somewhat unsteadily by.

"We didn't do that to him," said Diethrich, who had seen the un-
concealed look on my face, that of a man standing in the carnival
midway and eyeing the poster promises of the freak show. "The
cortisone makes his face swell a little, but everything else he was born
with."

"What have the tests shown?"

"No rejection. None whatsoever."

Anicic, the Yugoslavian doctor, said, "The boy is incredible. He is
leading a completely normal life. I see him about once a week, but
when I went on holiday for a month, I didn't see him at all. The only
noticeable complication has been an elevated white blood cell count
after the tiring five-day trip back home to Yugoslavia from Texas."
Duson lives with his widowed mother and receives a special allotment
from Tito's government to help pay his medical expenses. He is a
national hero there.

"I think we'll be able to cut down the cortisone," said Diethrich.
"Maybe shrink his face a little."

We returned to the frontenis court and in the middle of a
stormy doubles match with the ball hurtling at the forward wall,

Duson entered the court and picked up a racket to join in. Speedy Zweibeck, a new DeBakey fellow just down from New York, stopped and asked Duson politely to move to a grassy area for spectators and watch. The child obeyed, but in a few minutes he was back, still wanting to join the surgeons at their game. "Look, kid," said Speedy, half-exasperated, "if you don't get off the court, we're going to take your heart back."

Duson wandered to the nearby trampoline and climbed onto it, bouncing tentatively at first, then shouting with glee as he sprang up and down, his swollen face dripping with honest, joyful perspiration. "I hope you sewed that heart in good, Diethrich," said Speedy.

Later, when my team was beaten at the frontenis game, I plunged into the pool and swam underwater as long as my breath would allow me, rejoicing in the coolness and languor of the depths. When I surfaced, someone jumped in beside me and laughed loudly. It was Duson. "We can swim together," he said, and the boy with the faded scar on his pigeon chest was suddenly nothing more than another youth reveling in the summer afternoon, wanting to be accepted as a human being, not a medical oddity. We took eight laps together, talking, shouting, splashing, using the palms of our hands to slap the water and shower those watching, with amazement, our exhibition.

As we dried ourselves with thick beach towels, Duson talked of his rock group. "It is called The Beatniks," he said, "and I am the leader. I wrote a song called 'The First Step on the Moon' and last week it was number one on all the charts in Yugoslavia." He grinned broadly, waiting for my nod of compliment.

"You could get the same noise," said Anicic, "by putting two cats, two dogs, and a screech owl in the recording studio." Duson stuck his thumb in his soda bottle and shook it and sprayed his doctor.

"He doesn't like my music," said Duson, "but everybody else does. I make money to go to musical school." He was in his first year of a four-year musical education. He could look ahead that far!

Diethrich grilled hamburgers and hot dogs in the twilight and his star guest heaped a plate full with beans, potato salad, tomatoes, and pickles. He ate ravenously and stretched out on a horizontal deck chair. He belched and patted his stomach. When Diethrich walked by to get some more meat patties, Duson stopped him shyly and touched his arm. "Thank you," the boy said.

As the boy and his doctor took their leave, I shook their hands.

"I'm glad to see you don't favor your new heart," I said to my swimming partner.

"Days, sometimes weeks go by and I don't even think about it," he said. "I don't think about it today at all. . . ."

Despite the extraordinary witness born by Duson Vlaco, the heart-transplant program, completely moribund at St. Luke's Hospital, was scarcely more alive at Methodist. Howard Stapler's heart failure was treated by the cardiologists on DeBakey's staff and he recovered sufficiently to return to his Western novels, his home in Indiana, and yearnings for another heart. Twice again in the summer and autumn of 1970 he would fly back to Houston seemingly in the throes of death, only to be revived by medication and observation. He asked both Diethrich and DeBakey regularly when they were going to transplant him, but the answers he got were guarded and noncommital. Diethrich said the transplant program was blocked by lack of money, which was, in a large sense, true. Transplants had cost an average of $75,000 and a considerable portion had come from Baylor's research funds. In the inflation of Nixon's administration, money for medical research had grown increasingly scarce and there was no willingness on DeBakey's part to spend what there was on heart transplants.

Privately, the junior surgeons believed DeBakey to be totally disenchanted by the transplant experience. Cooley's record of 100 percent mortality, the unpleasantness of the artificial-heart trial, the enormous drain on the talents and capacities of the hospital staff in caring for transplant patients, and the public's disinterest in donating hearts had brewed a bitter potion. "The Professor's career has been built on winning," said one of the younger men. "Why risk failure this late in his game?"

In late August, Ted Diethrich summoned his courage, rehearsed mentally for the twelfth time what he would say, and asked DeBakey for a private audience. He spoke quickly and enthusiastically, looking directly into the magnified eyes behind the thick glasses. He would be resigning, Diethrich said. He had been privately working on a dream to build his own heart institute, and now it was far enough along to be assured. "I'm going to Phoenix, Arizona," Diethrich said. He had found backers to build a $3 million addition to an existing Catholic hospital. He would form his own team of cardiologists, nurses, and pump technicians and there would be affiliations with the University of Arizona Medical School.

"Where is that?" asked DeBakey.

"In Tucson, about 150 miles away."

"That's about close enough," said DeBakey wearily, caught up at that moment in a struggle across the street with the Baylor faculty over his plan to slice one year from the four-year medical education and, hopefully, turn out doctors faster.

DeBakey did not attempt to dissuade his junior man, even though Diethrich was an invaluable member of his team, even though the Arizona Heart Institute, if successful, would service a portion of the country, the American Southwest, which had sent hundreds of patients to Houston. "Keep me informed," was all he said.

With the long-kept-quiet cat finally out of the bag, Diethrich spoke with excitement as he began recruiting. "It's going to be FAN-TAS-TIC," he fairly cried. "Suppose a doctor calls up and says, 'I've got a 45-year-old man who's just had an acute coronary, what can we do for him?' Well, the Arizona Heart Institute will have on hand a 24-hour-a-day ambulance with a doctor inside. They go out, bring this man in, *not* to the emergency room of a hospital, but to an area in our Institute that is equipped for everything from minor IV support to coronary catheterization to immediate bypass surgery. Nobody has this concept yet. This is the Outer Space Medicine of the '70s, of the '80s. We can pick up patients by helicopter from 200 miles around. We'll have our own jet, too. When somebody calls in sick from Chicago, what can we do for him? We can do many things for him, we can send our jet out to get him and perhaps save his life. . . . The philosophy of so many doctors is twenty years back—a hundred years back. They give a heart-attack victim an EKG, put him to bed, start him on exercise. I'm not at all sure that you shouldn't start exploring his vessels right away, do cardiac catheterization *immediately* upon his arrival at the hospital. We have surgical methods now to *immediately* revascularize the heart, to *immediately* restore a new blood supply. If you look at statistics on coronary death rate of people admitted to hospitals who have low blood pressure on arrival, 75 percent of them never leave the hospital. This doesn't even take into consideration the 50 percent who never even arrive.

"These may seem like wild, far-out ideas, but these are things I could never develop here in Houston. There's no way for me to do this in Houston. I've got to put myself in a position where I have my own team. And I can't sit around another five or ten years until DeBakey retires. When he leaves, there's going to be the maddest scramble for power you ever saw. . . . We're going to start clean in Arizona. I'm going to have only people who can get excited. People that you can't excite, I'm through with. I've got to have people beside me whom you can light a bomb under and they're in orbit—seven days a week. I want a handful of people with me who can change the world of heart care."

Don Bricker had said there were a half-dozen DeBakeys. A year after *L'affaire Cooley*, there seemed to be a hundred more, all possessed, consumed, *driven* to plant footprints so large that no new wave could wash them away. There was the DeBakey boldly seeking $30 million for Baylor in a recession year, the DeBakey overhauling the medical school's curriculum and doubling the freshman class enrollment from 84 to 168 and doing it on a few weeks' notice over the anguished objection of more than one veteran faculty member. There was the DeBakey flying as commuter to Washington and meeting with Senator Edward Kennedy to write a universal health-plan bill that would, as one Houston doctor complained, "push American medicine totally over the brink into the swamp of socialism." DeBakey snapped back to all such attacks that medical care in his country was a right, not a privilege, that it belonged to all Americans, not only those over 65. There was the DeBakey wooing in person and on telephone some of the great names in science, attempting to persuade them to come to Houston to fill five long-vacant academic chairs at Baylor—vacant, some said, because the great names did not relish working within the volcano of Mike DeBakey. There was the DeBakey pushing *his* artificial heart program with a new man down to head it, wrapping it in security measures comparable to a NASA installation. There was even the DeBakey appearing on midnight television talk shows, giving awards of merit to Jerry

Lewis. But these were only the public DeBakeys. The private one was buried even deeper in a body of secrecy. He had placed himself within a labyrinth to which all access seemed blocked. Suspicion appeared to emanate from him toward all. "I can understand how Mike is hurt over the artificial heart," said one who had known him for years, "but I cannot understand why he has to distrust practically everybody in the Medical Center."

He withdrew more and more to the locked office, preferring more and more the sureness of the telephone over the permanence of the letter. The only man whom he could fully trust was Michael E. DeBakey. The only man to fully understand what he would do, his wrath, his wisdom, his loneliness, was Michael E. DeBakey.

Geoff, the expelled surgical resident, was reinstated as abruptly as he had been thrown out. He never learned the exact reason for his dramatic censure and expulsion from the hospital, nor did he know why DeBakey casually invited him back into the program, with credit for the academic year, with an even better job in the Ben Taub charity program. Only DeBakey knew.

Though he was increasingly engaged on matters academic and national, the senior surgeon did not short his responsibilities in the operating room. There his manner and disposition had not changed. Toward the end of August, 1970, there were two vivid examples.

The first case was a Tetralogy of Fallot, a boy who had flown from Europe with money raised by his village. "Mike is always interested in these mercy-flight cases," said a junior surgeon as he recounted the story. "Anyway, the kid had the usual VSD, which we sewed up, but we couldn't get the boy off the pump. We tried for 30 minutes and DeBakey was distraught. He was, in fact, going out of his mind. He yelled for another anesthesiologist to come into the room, and when he did, and when *that* didn't help, Mike cried, 'It must be metabolic,' and he called for a new cardiologist. All the time he was crying, 'Do something! Do something!' When nothing worked, when every new idea had been exhausted, Mike and the assisting surgeon discovered what had really happened. The kid's aorta was coming out of the right side of the heart, a freaky thing. We had fixed one defect but overlooked the other more complex problem, which was uncorrectable from the beginning. The kid died and Mike looked up with his eyes glistening and said, 'Who's going to go out there and tell that mother her child is dead?'"

The one DeBakey practice that most annoyed his young surgeons was his custom of making out the surgical schedule himself, not permitting it to be done by anyone else. "Consequently," griped a junior surgeon, "you don't know who you're going to operate on tomorrow until nine or ten the night before. The blood bank has to spend all night rushing around and calling to locate blood, and anesthesia has to wait until 10 P.M. to talk to the patients, and nobody gets much sleep. But that's the way Mike does things."

On a Sunday night, after having been out of town for a few days, DeBakey made rounds and scheduled a staggering array of operations for Monday morning—eleven in all, including four coronary bypasses and one gasendarterectomy, those new, meticulous procedures that gossip held DeBakey had not learned. Or perhaps *could* not do. On the Monday morning, as he scrubbed in at seven, DeBakey frowned upon hearing that George Noon was on vacation. There were some who later claimed that DeBakey knew it all along. For what was about to happen would be talked about in Houston medicine for years to come.

His face grew more stormy when Ted Diethrich did but one case, a carotid—reaming out of the carotid artery is always done first because such cases are normally easy and gotten out of the way quickly—and then flew off to New York to deliver a paper to a medical meeting. There were some who later claimed that DeBakey knew of Diethrich's trip as well.

"Nobody wants to work any more," griped DeBakey as he began a coronary artery bypass operation at eleven, the procedure that Denton Cooley was now committed to and proclaiming its beauty at medical meetings. The operation took two grueling hours with the tenseness on DeBakey's face apparent to everyone in the room. When he was done, it was early afternoon, and the staff assumed he would do perhaps one more case and cancel the schedule until his assisting surgeons returned. But instead he moved wordlessly to the adjoining operating room and began a valve replacement. By 4 P.M. it became obvious something was up. At six, the nurses and junior men began eyeing the operating room clock because it was known that DeBakey had a 10 P.M. flight to Washington and he would have to quit by eight to make it. His temper had flashed so often during the day that no one dared ask if he was going to the airport. Once during the long afternoon he had exclaimed that he was in the company of incompetents and that he would do all the work himself. He tried to hold the retractor, the sucking machine, and the sewing needle all at once. "If I only had three hands," he cried out, "I could operate all by myself. . . ."

Between early-evening cases, he slipped out and made rounds with a nurse. He also sent out for hamburgers to feed the entire team, an act of kindness that startled the newer members. He moved back and forth from operating rooms 2 to 3 to 4 as the cases were brought in. He would let one of the assistants make the opening skin incision, but that was all. "God help us," murmured one of the residents as the evening began, "he's going to do the whole schedule." DeBakey's work, that of three surgeons, was breathtaking. Eight o'clock came and went, nine flew by, and at ten one of the strong young doctors who starred each Sunday at Ted Deithrich's sports marathons felt the pain in his spine and the heaviness in his eyes, but he remained spellbound by the power and beauty of DeBakey's surgery.

At midnight, the senior surgeon called for the gasendarterectomy patient who was fetched somewhat bewildered from his room and wheeled to the operating room. There DeBakey, with no sign of weariness, began his eleventh operation of the day, a day which had begun at 7 A.M. He made the tiny incision within the artery of the heart and injected the whiffs of carbon dioxide to loosen the layers of occlusion, those layers which threatened to close the artery and possibly bring on a heart attack. With grace and sureness he loosened the core and pulled it out, holding the offending mass for a moment in the strong lights from the four spots that bathed him and the patient's heart. "He was the tallest man I ever saw," said Speedy Zweibeck when it was over, "and the proudest, and certainly the youngest."

When he was done sewing up the eleventh and last patient of a day that had stretched eighteen and a half unbroken hours, DeBakey glanced up at the operating room clock and saw that it was 1:25 A.M. Around him stood men and women, who, had they not been masked and gowned and gloved, would have applauded and shook his hand. Someone else could play the concerto well in Houston. DeBakey was exhilarated as he walked to the heavy swinging doors. He opened one as if to leave. Instead he stuck his head out and he cried in a voice of triumph that burst through his mask and broke the quietness of the empty corridor: "Anybody else out there want an operation?"

Summary of Heart Transplants as of March 1, 1971

Total No. of Transplants: 170
      U.S.   :   108
      Foreign: 62

Total No. of Recipients: 167
Total No. of Deaths: 143
Number of Survivors: 24
      U.S.   :   18
      Foreign: 6
Total Number of Countries: 20
Total Number of Surgical Teams: 65
      U.S.   :   29
      Foreign: 36

Survivors as of Mar. 1, 1971	Date of Surgery	Days Surviving
Russell	8-24-68	919
Carroll	8-31-68	912
Vlaco	9-18-68	894
Sanchez	10-01-68	881
Anick	10-21-68	861
Sheaffer	10-26-68	856
Parkinson	11-03-68	848
Johnston	11-17-68	834
Vitira	11-27-68	824
Kaminski	12-01-68	820
Gilian	2-08-69	751
Pounds	4-14-69	686
Fisher	4-17-69	683
Trout	5-22-69	648
Paul	8-13-69	565
Johnson	9-03-69	544
Bartholomew	9-29-69	518
Van Buren	1-04-70	421
Marshall	1-16-70	409
Madigan	4-28-70	307
Townswick	7-04-70	240
Cope	10-15-70	137
Kinsley	1-11-71	48
Knudson	2-24-71	5

Human Heart Transplants *

Date of Transplant	Status †	Recipient/Donor	Age	Sex	Reported Cause of Death	Surgeon/Institution City, State, Country
01-23-64	Dead 2 hrs. 01-23-64	Unidentified Donor-Chimp	68 —	M —	heart too small	Hardy, University of Mississippi
12-3-67	Dead 18 ds.‡ 12-21-67	Washkansky Donor-Human	53 25	M M	infection/rejection	Barnard, Groote Schuur Hosp., Cape-town, South Africa
12-6-67	Dead 6½ hrs. 12-6-67	Baby Donor-Human	17 ds. 2 ds.	M M	metabolic and respiratory acidosis	Kantrowitz, Maimonides Hosp., Brooklyn, New York
01-2-68	Dead 593 ds. 8-17-69	Blaiberg Donor-Human	58 24	M M	chronic rejection	Barnard, Groote Schuur Hosp., Cape-town, South Africa
01-6-68	Dead 15 ds. 1-21-68	Kasperak Donor-Human	57 43	M M	internal hemorrhage	Shumway, Stanford Med. Ctr., Palo Alto, California
01-10-68	Dead 8½ hr. 1-10-68	Block Donor-Human	58 29	M F	left ventricular failure	Kantrowitz, Maimonides Hospital

* Office of Heart Information, The National Heart Institute. † Status—time survived. ‡ Ds.—days survived.

Date	Recipient / Donor	Age	Sex	Cause of death	Surgeon, Hospital	Outcome
02-16-68	*Chithan* Donor–Human	27 / 20	M / F	pulmonary hypertension	P. K. Sen, King Edward Hosp., Bombay, India	Dead 3 hr. 2-17-68
04-27-68	*Roblain* Donor–Human	66 / 23	M / M	embolism / brain damage	Cabrol, La Petie, Paris, France	Dead 2 ds. 4-29-68
05-2-68	*Rizor* Donor–Human	40 / 43	M / M	deprivation of oxygen / pulmonary embolism	Shumway, Stanford Med. Ctr.	Dead 3½ ds. 5-6-68
05-3-68	*Thomas* Donor–Human	47 / 15	M / F	rejection	D. Cooley, St. Luke's Hosp., Houston, Texas	Dead 204 ds. 11-23-68 (Note: this patient received a second transplant 11/18/68)
05-3-68	*West* Donor–Human	45 / 26	M / M	multiple pulmonary emboli	Longmore, National Heart Hosp., London, England	Dead 45 ds. 6-17-68
05-5-68	*Cobb* Donor–Human	48 / 15	M / M	leukopenia, pneumonia, and sepsis	Cooley, St. Luke's	Dead 3 ds. 5-8-68
05-7-68	*Stuckwish* Donor–Human	62 / 36	M / M	renal and hepatic failure	Cooley, St. Luke's	Dead 7 ds. 5-14-68
05-8-68	*Reynes* Donor–Human	65 / 35	M / M	pulmonary injury, cerebral air embolism	Negre, St. Eloi Hosp., Mt. Pelier, France	Dead 2 ds. 5-10-68

Human Heart Transplants (Cont'd.)

Date of Transplant	Status	Recipient/ Donor	Age	Sex	Reported Cause of Death	Surgeon/Institution City, State, Country
05-12-68	Dead 523 ds. 10-17-69	*Boulogne* Donor–Human	56 39	M M	rejection	Charles DuBost, Broussais Hosp., Paris, France
05-21-68	Dead 146 ds. 10-14-68	*Fierro* Donor–Human	54 17	M M	cardiac arrest/rejection	Cooley, St. Luke's
05-25-68	Dead 7 ds. 6-1-68	*Klett* Donor–Human	53 48	M M	total rejection	Richard Lower, Med. College of Virginia, Richmond, Va.
05-26-68	Dead 28 ds. 6-23-68	*F. da Cunha* Donor–Human	24 40	M M	rejection	E. Zerbini, Hosp. das Clinicas, Brazil
05-31-68	Dead 5 ds. 6-5-68	*A. Serrano* Donor–Human	54 47	M M	cerebral embolism	Miguel Bellizzi, Clinic Lanus, Buenos Aires, Argentina
05-31-68	Dead 1 day 6-1-68	*A. Murphy* Donor–Human	59 38	M F	low-output heart failure	Pierre Grondin, Montreal Heart Institute, Canada
05-31-68	Dead 0 hrs. 5-31-68	*R. Smith* Donor–Human	39 29	M M	malfunction of right ventricle	C. W. Lillehei, Cornell Medical Center, NYC

Date	Recipient/Status	Age	Sex	Cause of death	Surgeon, Hospital
06-7-68	Dead 1½ hrs. *E. Matthews* 6-7-68 / Donor-Human	41 / 26	F / M	acute rejection	Webb, U. of Texas Southwestern Med. School, Dallas, Texas / Cooley, St. Luke's
06-12-68	*Willoughby* 06-12-68 / Sheep (125 lbs.)	48 / –	M / –	heart did not start	Cooley, St. Luke's
06-28-68	Dead 156 ds. *Paris* 12-1-68 / Donor-Human	49 / 23	M / M	asphyxiation following indigestion	Grondin, Montreal Heart Institute
06-28-68	Dead 133 ds. *Penaloza* 11-8-68 / Donor-Human	24 / 32	F / M	cerebral embolus	J. Kaplan, Admiral Neff Naval Hosp., Valparaiso, Chile
07-2-68	Dead 0 hrs. *Z.M.* 7-2-68 / Calf heart	14 / –	F / –	?	Poznan City Hosp., Warsaw, Poland
07-2-68	Dead 149 ds. *DeBord* 11-28-68 / Donor-Human	48 / 50	M / M	chronic rejection	Cooley, St. Luke's
07-9-68	Dead 5 hrs. *Horvathona* 7-9-68 / Donor-Human	49 / 46	F / M	?	Siska, Bratislava Univ. Hosp., Prague, Czechoslovakia
07-20-68	Dead 266 ds. *Everman* 4-12-69 / Donor-Human	58 / 33	M / F	probably arrhythmias	Cooley, St. Luke's
07-23-68	Dead 170 ds. *Jurgens* 1-9-69 / Donor-Human	57 / 16	M / M	chronic rejection	Cooley, St. Luke's
07-26-68	Dead 2 ds. *Forde* 7-28-68 / Donor-Human	47 / 34	M / M	ventricular failure	Longmore, National Heart Hosp., London, England

Human Heart Transplants (Cont'd.)

Date of Transplant	Status	Recipient/ Donor	Age	Sex	Reported Cause of Death	Surgeon/Institution City, State, Country
07-29-68	Dead 56 ds. 9-23-68	*Brunk* Donor–Human	49 40	F F	sepsis, GI hemorrhage, thrombocytopenia	Cooley, St. Luke's
08-8-68	Dead 82 ds. 10-29-68	*Miyazaki* Donor–Human	18 21	M M	acute respiratory infection	Juro Wada, Sapproro Hosp., Japan
08-18-68	Dead 7 ds. 8-25-68	*M. Giannaris* Donor–Human	5 11	F M	cardiac arrest/ acute rejection	Cooley, St. Luke's
8-19-68	Dead 68 ds. 10-26-68	*Van Bates* Donor–Human	50 37	M F	herpes sepsis, pneumonia	Cooley, St. Luke's
8-22-68	Dead 46 ds. 10-8-68	*Drake* Donor–Human	43 21	M M	pneumonia	Shumway, Stanford
8-24-68	Surviving	Donor–Human *Russell*	43 17	M M		Lower, Medical College of Virginia
8-30-68	Dead 11 ds. 9-10-68	*Zaor* Donor–Human	58 35	M M	stroke	Grondin, Montreal Heart Institute
8-31-68	Dead 624 ds. 5-17-70	*McKee* Donor–Human	50 39	M M	?	Shumway, Stanford

Date	Status	Recipient / Donor	Age	Sex	Cause	Surgeon / Hospital
8-31-68	Surviving	Carroll / Donor-Human	50 / 20	M / F		Michael E. DeBakey, Houston Methodist Hospital
9-1-68	Dead 443 ds. 11-18-69	Anolik / Donor-Human	46 / 22	M / M	rejection	H. Bahnson, Presbyterian U. Hosp., Pittsburgh, Pa.
9-2-68	Dead 409 ds. 10-16-69	U. Orlandi / Donor-Human	48 / 39	M / M	rejection	Zerbini, Das Clinicas, Sao Paulo, Brazil
9-4-68	Dead 476 ds. 12-24-69	Lawson / Donor-Human	50 / 25	M / F	acute M.I.; chronic rejection	D. B. Effler, Cleveland Clinic
9-5-68	Dead 8 ds. 9-13-68	Singleton / Donor-Human	47 / 17	M / M	cardiac arrest	DeBakey, Houston Methodist
9-8-68	Dead 621 ds. 5-21-70	Smith / Donor-Human	52 / 36	M / F	cancer of stomach	Barnard, Groote Schuur Hospital
9-10-68	Dead 132 ds. 1-20-69	Asche / Donor-Human	48 / 27	F / M	hepatitis	Shumway, Stanford
9-11-68	Dead 117 ds. 1-6-69	R. Brien / Donor-Human	58 / 16	M / M	pulmonary infarction	Grondin, Montreal Heart Institute, Canada
9-13-68	Dead 14 hrs. 9-13-68	Pardesi / Donor-Human	21 / 25	M / F	renal failure	Sen, Bombay, India

Human Heart Transplants (Cont'd.)

Date of Transplant	Status	Recipient/ Donor	Age	Sex	Reported Cause of Death	Surgeon/Institution City, State, Country
9-15-68	Dead 111 ds. 1-4-69	Lanning Donor-Human	52 20	M M	monelia brain abscess	T. E. Starzl, U. of Colo. Med. Ctr., Denver
9-15-68	Dead 14 hrs. 9-16-68	Lee Donor-Human	2 mos. 1 da.	F F	pulmonary insufficiency	Cooley, St. Luke's
9-17-68	Dead 2 ds. 9-19-68	Grille Donor-Human	44 46	M M	acute kidney insufficiency	C. Martinez Bordiu, La Paz Clinic, Madrid, Spain
09-18-68	Dead 6 hrs. 9-18-68	Sabisan Donor-Human	45 27	M F	irreversible ventricular fibrillation	J. M. Rocha, Central Military Hosp., Caracas, Venezuela
09-18-68	Surviving	Vlaco Donor-Human	16 36	M M		DeBakey, Houston Methodist
09-18-68	Dead 62 ds. 11-19-68	Desriviers, M. Donor-Human	51 19	M M	herpes viremia and cerebral pseudomonas abscess	Grondin, Montreal Heart Institute
09-19-68	Dead 88 ds. 12-16-68	Pfohl Donor-Human	57 46	M M	lung infection	DeBakey, Houston Methodist

Date	Status	Recipient / Donor	Age	Sex	Cause of death	Surgeon / Hospital
09-20-68	Dead 446 ds. 12-10-69	*Barnum* / Donor-Human	50 / 37	M / M	pneumonia	D. Kahn, U. of Michigan Medical Center
09-23-68	Dead 22 ds. 10-15-68	*Martin* / Donor-Human	46 / 17	M / M	cardiac arrest	DeBakey, Houston Methodist
10-1-68	Surviving	*N.O. Sanchez* / Donor-Human	21 / 17	M / M		J. Kaplan, Admiral Neff Naval Hospital, Chile
10-2-68	Dead 5 ds. 10-7-68	*Pratt* / Donor-Human	46 / 43	M / M	acute rejection	Webb, U. of Texas S.W. Medical School, Dallas
10-5-68	Dead 61 ds. 12-5-68	*Larson* / Donor-Human	54 / 28	F / F	pneumonia	Shumway, Stanford
10-9-68	Dead 204 ds. 5-1-69	*P. Ongaro* / Donor-Human	42 / 33	M / M	rejection	Donald Wilson, Toronto Western Hospital
10-12-68	Dead 157 ds. 3-18-69	*M. Schmidt* / Donor-Human	54 / 28	F / F	bowel perforation	DeBakey, Methodist Hospital
10-15-68	Dead 15 hrs. 10-16-68	*Bernardez* / Donor-Human	19 / 35	F / M	complication in blood coagulation	Bellizzi, Model Clinic, Buenos Aires, Argentina
10-18-68	Dead 177 ds. 4-13-69	*Harrison* / Donor-Human	50 / 20	M / M	ruptured colon	DeBakey, Methodist Hosp.

Human Heart Transplants (Cont'd.)

Date of Transplant	Status	Recipient/ Donor	Age	Sex	Reported Cause of Death	Surgeon/Institution City, State, Country
10-20-68	Dead 60 ds. 12-19-68	*Y. Therrien* Donor-Human	45 20	F M	acute rejection crisis	Grondin, Montreal Heart Institute
10-21-68	Surviving	*Anick* Donor-Human	49 30	F M		D. Lepley, Jr., Milwaukee St. Luke's Hosp., Wisconsin
10-23-68	Dead 45 ds. 12-7-68	*Pye* Donor-Human	57 30	M M	hemorrhage following surgical complications	Harry Windsor, St. Vincent's Hosp. Sydney, Australia
10-23-68	Dead 7 ds. 10-30-68	*Johnson* Donor-Human	19 19	F M	acute rejection	Lower, Medical Col. of Va.
10-24-68	Dead 6 hrs. 10-24-68	*Capobianco* Donor-Human	42 41	M F	cardiac arrest	DeBakey, Methodist Hosp.
10-25-68	Dead 126 ds. 2-28-69	*J. Decker* Donor-Human	52 49	M F	chronic rejection	Cooley, St. Luke's
10-25-68	Dead 54 ds. 12-18-68	*L. Senechal* Donor-Human	35 25	M M	rejection	Grondin, Montreal Heart Institute
10-26-68	Surviving	*Sheaffer* Donor-Human	54 20	M ?		Shumway, Stanford

Date	Status	Patient	Age	Sex	Cause of death	Surgeon / Hospital
10-29-68	Dead 9 ds. 11-7-68	H. Taylor	45	M	pneumonia/infection	D. Wilson, Toronto Western
		Donor-Human	20	M		
10-30-68	Dead 18 ds. 11-17-68	Starcher	23	M	rejection	Lower, Med. College of Virginia
		Donor-Human	24	M		
11-3-68	Dead 4 ds. 11-7-68	Cumbie	40	M	failure of liver/kidneys	DeBakey, Methodist Hosp.
		Donor-Human	42	M		
11-3-68	Surviving	Parkinson	52	M		L. MacLean, Royal Victoria Hosp., Montreal, Canada
		Donor-Human	28	F		
11-5-68	Dead 7 ds. 11-12-68	Lebowitz	50	M	rejection	Cooley, St. Luke's
		Donor-Human	27	M		
11-5-68	Dead 1 day 11-6-68	Unidentified	25	F	acute rejection	Alexandar Vishnevsky, Leningrad, Russia
		Donor-Human	19	M		
11-9-68	Dead 47 ds. 12-26-68	Perbacs	55	M	bacterial pneumonia	Cooley, St. Luke's
		Donor-Human	27	F		
11-11-68	Dead 38 ds. 12-19-68	A. Martine	44	M	acute rejection	Grondin, Montreal Heart
		Donor-Human	15	M		
11-11-68	Dead 13 ds. 11-24-68	Moissonier	34	M	acute rejection	Pierre Michaud, Edouward Harriot Hosp, Lyons, France
		Donor-Human	50	M		
11-13-68	Dead 7 ds. 11-20-68	Gagnier	54	M	cerebral embolism	W. G. Bigelow, Toronto Gen. Hosp., Canada
		Donor-Human	22	M		

Human Heart Transplants (Cont'd.)

Date of Transplant	Status	Recipient/ Donor	Age	Sex	Reported Cause of Death	Surgeon/Institution City, State, Country
11-13-68	Dead 14 hrs. 11-14-68	*Wippler* Donor-Human	44 44	M M	ventricular fibrillation	Ken Morris, Melbourne, Australia
11-16-68	Dead 498 ds. 3-29-70	*Boyd* Donor-Human	50 38	M F	pneumonia/rejection	Cooley, St. Luke's
11-17-68	Dead 40 ds. 12-27-68	*Henon* Donor-Human	53 50	M F	rejection	Guilmet, Foch Hospital, Paris
11-17-68	Surviving	*P. Johnston* Donor-Human	54 18	M M		C. Baker, St. Michael's Hosp., Toronto, Canada
11-20-68	Dead 3 ds. 11-23-68 (Note: received a second transplant 11/20/68)	*Hammerly* Donor-Human	56 ?	M ?	stroke	Shumway, Stanford
11-20-68	Dead 3 ds. 11-23-68 (Note: received first transplant 5/3/68. Survived a total of 202 days. A total of 3 days from date of second transplant.)	*Thomas* Donor-Human	47 47	M F	cardiac failure/ rejection	Cooley, St. Luke's
11-22-68	Dead 281 ds. 8-30-69	*Karraker* Donor-Human	49 ?	M ?	irregular heart action	Shumway, Stanford

Date	Outcome	Recipient / Donor	Age	Sex	Cause	Surgeon, Hospital
11-22-68	Dead 3 hrs. 11-22-68	D. R. Onato / Donor–Human	30 / 14	F / M	?	Kaplan, Chile
11-22-68	Dead 18 hrs. 11-22-68	Karazog / Donor–Human	33 / 18	F / M	liver ceased functioning, failure of blood to clot	Kemal Bayazit, Yuksek Ihtias Hosp., Ankara, Turkey
11-24-68	Dead 14 hrs. 11-24-68	Mal Veaux / Donor–Human	37 / 47	M / M	irreversible kidney failure	Binet, Marie Lannelongue Hospital, Paris, France
11-24-68	Dead 400 ds. 12-29-69	Fores / Donor–Human	48 / 46	M / M	rejection	DuBost, Broussais Hosp., Paris
11-25-68	Dead 1 day 11-26-68	Akgul / Donor–Human	26 / 50	M / M	cardiac insufficiency	S. Ersek, Istanbul, Turkey, Haydarpasa Chest Surgery Ctr.
11-25-68	Dead 70 ds. 2-3-69	S. Seidenberg / Donor–Human	56 / 26	M / M	rejection	Vincent L. Gott, Johns Hopkins Hosp., Baltimore, Maryland
11-26-68	Dead 20 hrs. 11-27-68	Mazzega / Donor–Human	56 / 33	M / M	cardiac arrest	DuBost, Broussais Hosp., Paris
11-27-68	Surviving	Vitira / Donor–Human	48 / 25	M / M		E. Henry, Jules Cantini Cardio. Med. Ctr., Marseilles, France

Human Heart Transplants (Cont'd.)

Date of Transplant	Status	Recipient/ Donor	Age	Sex	Reported Cause of Death	Surgeon/Institution City, State, Country
11-29-68	Dead 13 ds. 12-12-68	*Wackstein* Donor-Human	54 40	M M	rejection	Cooley, St. Luke's
11-29-68	Dead 105 ds. 3-14-69	*G. Levesque* Donor-Human	54 23	M M	cerebral thrombosis	Grondin, Montreal Heart Institute
12-1-68	Surviving	*Kaminski* Donor-Human	38 22	M M		Kahn, U. of Michigan Med. Ctr., Ann Arbor, Michigan
12-5-68	Dead 14 ds. 12-19-68	*Y. Sulam* Donor-Human	43 ?.	M M	kidney failure/ pneumonia/rejection	M. Levy, Bellinson Hosp., Petah Tikva, Israel
12-16-68	Dead 43 ds. 1-28-69	*Julliard* Donor-Human	22 21	M M	congestive heart failure	Effler, Cleveland Clinic
12-22-68	Dead 225 ds. 8-4-69	*Marion* Donor-Human	28 30	M M	?	F. Fontan, Tondu Hosp., Bordeaux, France
12-25-68	Dead 5 hrs. 12-25-68	*Whippie* Donor-Human	8 da. 2 da.	M M	cardiac failure	C. F. Kittle, U. of Chicago Billings Hospital

Date	Outcome	Recipient/Donor	Age	Sex	Cause	Surgeon, Hospital
12-27-68	Dead 91 ds. 3-28-69	E. Cramer / Donor-Human	50 / 24	M / M	rejection	Hassan Najafi, Presbyterian St. Luke's, Chicago, Ill.
01-1-69	Dead 114 ds. 4-25-69	Alderblum / Donor-Human	64 / 48	M / M	acute rejection	C. W. Lillehei, Cornell Med. Ctr., NYC
01-4-69	Dead 0 hrs. 1-4-69	Tomaszewski / Donor-Human	35 / 26	M / M	right ventricular hypertension	Jan Moll, Lodz Medical Acad., Warsaw, Poland
01-5-69	Dead 37 ds. 2-11-69	Chancey / Donor-Human	59 / 14	M / M	rejection	DeBakey, Methodist Hosp.
01-5-69	Dead 7 ds. 1-12-69	Giordano / Donor-Human	44 / 54	M / ?	pulmonary hypertension/myopathy	Lillehei, Cornell Medical Center
01-6-69	Dead 7 ds. 1-13-69	Whitten / Donor-Human	49 / 44	M / M	brain hemorrhage/pneumonia	Hardy, Univ. of Mississipi Medical Center
01-6-69	Dead 83 ds. 3-30-69	C. Praca / Donor-Human	52 / 28	M / M	pulmonary embolus	Zerbini, Das Clinicas, Brazil
01-17-69	Dead 4 hrs. 1-17-69	Evans / Donor-Human	49 / 38	M / M	progressive pulmonary hypertension	W. E. Neville, VA Hospital, Hines, Illinois
01-23-69	Dead 2 ds. 1-25-69	Wolfram / Donor-Human	47 / 13	M / M	brain damage/edema of brain	G. J. Magovern, Allegheny Gen. Hosp., Pittsburgh, Pa.

Human Heart Transplants (Cont'd.)

Date of Transplant	Status	Recipient/ Donor	Age	Sex	Reported Cause of Death	Surgeon/Institution City, State, Country
2-8-69	Dead 30 ds. 3-10-69	*Corbn* Donor-Human	7 8	F M	lung infection/ rejection	James Helmsworth, Children's Hospital, Cincinnatti, Ohio
2-8-69	Surviving	*S. Gilien* Donor-Human	43 ?	M ?		Shumway, Stanford
2-13-69	Dead 1 day 2-14-69	*Zebner* Donor-Human	36 39	M F	traumatic coronary thrombosis pre- transplant	Sebening, Univ. Clinic Munich, Germany
2-15-69	Dead 10 ds. 2-25-69	*D. Allan* Donor-Human	55 24	M M	rejection	Shumway, Stanford
2-20-69·	Dead 64 ds. 4-25-69	*J. Hansel* Donor-Human	36 57	M M	rejection	Lillehei, Cornell
2-20-69	Dead 41 ds. 4-2-69	*R. Newell* Donor-Human	58 23	M F	hemorragic pneumonitis	R. J. Cleveland, Harbor Gen. Hosp., Torrance, California
3-4-69	Dead 99 ds. 6-11-69	*I. Morris* Donor-Human	56 26	M M	hepatitis	Cooley, St. Luke's

Date	Status	Patient / Donor	Age	Sex	Cause	Surgeon, Location
3-16-69	Dead 1-29-70 (Note: re-transplanted 1-16-70)	G. Rector Donor-Human	43 24	M M	survived 306 ds. with 1st trans.	Kahn, University Hospital, Ann Harbor, Michigan
3-22-69	Dead 1 day 3-23-69	W. Hanus Donor-Human	38 28	M M	cardiac arrest	Sebening, Univ. Clinic, Munich, Germany
3-29-69	Dead 39 ds. 5-7-69	G. Campbell Donor-Human	42 ?	M ?	?	Shumway, Stanford
04-3-69	Dead 5 ds. 4-8-69	D. Schmidt Donor-Human	40 ?	F ?	rejection/hepsis	Lillehei, NY Hospital
*04-4-69	Re-transplanted 4-7-69	H. Karp Received a total artificial heart replacement (63 hrs.)	47	M		D. Cooley, St. Luke's
04-4-69	Dead 49 ds. 5-23-69	J. Washburn Donor-Human	35 41	M F	acute rejection	R. J. Baird, Toronto Western, Canada
04-7-69	Dead 1 day 4-8-69	H. Karp Donor-Human	47 40	M F	pseudomonis septicemia	D. Cooley, St. Luke's
04-7-69	Dead 64 ds. 6-10-69	W. Killops Donor-Human	63 43	M F	rejection	Barnard, South Africa
04-14-69	Dead 91 ds. 7-14-69	E. Hoffman Donor-Human	54 27	M M	unidentified infection	A. Senning, Zurich, Switzerland

Human Heart Transplants (Cont'd.)

Date of Transplant	Status	Recipient/ Donor	Age	Sex	Reported Cause of Death	Surgeon/Institution City, State, Country
04-14-69	Surviving	Pounds Donor-Human	58 20	M M		Shumway, Stanford
04-15-69	Dead 31 ds. 5-16-69	T. Chambers Donor-Human	44 30	M M	acute rejection	DeBakey, Methodist Houston
04-17-69	Surviving	D. Fisher Donor-Human	38 33	F M		Barnard, Groote. Schuur Hosp., Cape Town, South Africa
04-24-69	Dead 14 ds. 5-8-69	H. Goodkin Donor-Human	55 29	M F	parasitic pneumonia/ rejection	Gentsch, Miami Heart Inst., Miami Beach, Florida
04-26-69	Dead 6 ds. 5-2-69	M. Hand Donor-Human	35 35	M F	acute rejection	le Roux, Wentworth Hospital, Durban South Africa
05-11-69	Dead 35 ds. 6-15-69	Berg Donor-Human	48 16	M F	rejection	Lillehei, New York Hospital
05-16-69	Dead 107 ds. 8-31-69	C. Hendrick Donor-Human	59 29	M F	cardiac arrest	D. Ross, Guy's Hosp., London, England

Date	Status	Recipient / Donor	Age	Sex	Cause of death	Surgeon / Hospital
05-22-69	Surviving	R. Trout Donor-Human	34 ?	M ?		Shumway, Stanford
06-2-69	Dead 41 ds. 7-13-69	D.H. Halbeck Donor-Human	54 20	M M	rejection reaction	Angell, V.A. Hospital, Palo Alto, California
06-3-69	Dead 142 ds. 10-23-69	D.S. Marlow Donor-Human	52 25	M M	systemic infection	Cooley, St. Luke's
06-28-69	Dead 42 ds. 8-9-69	Munklewitz Donor-Human	56 32	M F	pneumonia/renal failure	Lillehei, New York Hospital
07-7-69	Dead 74 ds. 9-19-69	Bubler Donor-Human	46 28	M M	arrythmia	A. Senning, Clinic Kantonestital, Zurich, Switzerland
07-10-69	Dead 9 hrs. 7-10-69	H.L. Lutterbeck Donor-Human	46 31	M M	fibrinolysis and irreversible bleeding	E. Buechert, West End Hosp., Berlin, Germany
07-16-69	Dead 136 ds. 11-29-69	E.R. Wagenveld Donor-Human	52 ?	M ?	rejection	Shumway, Stanford
07-25-69	Dead 4 ds. 7-29-69	H. Wortman Donor-Human	59 17	M F	pulmonary emboli/renal failure	Lillehei, New York Hospital
07-28-69	Dead 5 ds. 8-2-69	B. Robinson Donor-Human	47 18	M M	pneumonia/renal failure	Lillehei, New York Hospital

HUMAN HEART TRANSPLANTS (Cont'd.)

DATE OF TRANSPLANT	STATUS	RECIPIENT/ DONOR	AGE	SEX	REPORTED CAUSE OF DEATH	SURGEON/INSTITUTION CITY, STATE, COUNTRY
08-13-69	Surviving	W. Paul Donor–Human	58 35	M M		Benson Roe, U. of California Med. Ctr., San Francisco, California
08-16-69	Dead 10 hrs. 8-16-69	H. Scales Donor–Human	54 ?	M ?	high blood pressure in lung causing lack of oxygen	Shumway, Stanford
09-3-69	Surviving	B. Johnson Donor–Human	45 ?	F ?		Shumway, Stanford
09-14-69	Dead 60 ds. 11-13-69	H. Joslyn Donor–Human	64 32	M M	?	Shumway, Stanford
09-25-69	Dead 26 ds. 10-21-69	H. Sims Donor–Human	54 41	M F	pneumonia	Cooley, St. Luke's
09-29-69	Surviving	Bartholomew Donor–Human	48 24	M M		Starzl, VA Hospital, Denver, Colorado
10-13-69	Dead 29 hrs. 10-15-69	D. Soltz Donor–Human	44 20	M M	?	le Roux, Wentworth Hosp., Durban, So. Africa

Date	Patient / Donor	Age	Sex	Cause	Surgeon / Hospital	Outcome
12-25-69	E. Falk / Donor-Human (also both lungs)	43 / 50	M / F	lung rejection/ pneumonia	Lillehei, New York Hospital	Dead 8 ds. 1-2-70
01-4-70	Van Buren / Donor-Human	40 / ?	M / ?		Shumway, Stanford	Surviving
01-8-70	Taylor / Donor-Human	52 / 36	M / F	massive respiratory infection	J. Ochsner, Ochsner Clinic, New Orleans, La.	Dead 116 ds. 5-4-70
01-13-70	Burke / Donor-Human	34 / ?	M / ?	rejection	DeBakey, Methodist Hosp., Houston, Texas	Dead 4 ds. 1-17-70
01-16-70	Rector / Donor-Human	44 / 24	M / M	kidney and liver failure	Kahn, University Hospital, Ann Arbor, Michigan	Dead 13 ds. (Note: See first trans. 3-16-69 306 ds. w/first heart)
01-16-70	Marshall / Donor-Human	49 / ?	M / ?		Shumway, Stanford	Surviving
02-10-70	W.N. Shepard / Donor-Human	49 / ?	M / F	rejection	Lower, Medical College of Virginia	Dead 58 ds. 4-13-70
04-18-70	L. Abbott / Donor-Human	54 / 43	M / M	heart could not function well	Kahn, U. of Michigan	Dead 0 hrs. 4-18-70

HUMAN HEART TRANSPLANTS (Cont'd.)

DATE OF TRANSPLANT	STATUS	RECIPIENT/ DONOR	AGE	SEX	REPORTED CAUSE OF DEATH	SURGEON/INSTITUTION CITY, STATE, COUNTRY
04-28-70	Surviving	*Madigan* Donor–Human	50 ?	M F	?	C. Baker, St. Michael's Hospital, Toronto, Canada
06-10-70	Dead 0 hrs. 5-10-70	*Beam* Donor–Human	41 ?	M ?	?	?, Stanford University
06-13-70	Dead 24 ds. 6-7-70	*Fillner* Donor–Human	37 45	F M	pancreas involvement	W. D. Johnson, St. Luke's, Milwaukee
06-13-70	Dead 47 ds. 6-29-70	*Wainwright* Donor–Human	62 ?	M ?	?	E. Stinson, Stanford
06-19-70	Dead 55 ds. 7-13-70	*Louderback* Donor–Human	49 ?	M ?	?	Shumway, Stanford
06-22-70	Dead 52 ds. 7-13-70	*McMahon* Donor–Human	50 ?	M ?	?	Shumway, Stanford
07-4-70	Surviving	*Townswick* Donor–Human	48 ?	M ?		Shumway, Stanford

07-21-70	Dead 45 ds. 9-4-70	*Robinson* Donor-Human	48 23	M M	?	?, University of Michigan
10-23-70	Dead 12 ds. 11-5-70	*Enzman* Donor-Human	21 ?	M ?	rejection	?, V.A. Hospital, Denver, Colorado

Bibliography

BOOKS

Bankoff, G., *The Story of Surgery*. London, Arthur Baker, Ltd., 1947.

Barnard, C. and Pepper, C. B., *One Life*. New York, Macmillan, 1970.

Blakeslee, Alton L. and Stamler, Jeremiah, *Your Heart Has Nine Lives: Nine Steps to Heart Health*. New York, Prentice-Hall, 1963.

Castiglioni, Arturo, *A History of Medicine*. Trans. by E. B. Krumbhaar. New York, Knopf, 1958.

Clark, R. L. and Cumley, R. W., *The Book of Health*. 2nd ed. Princeton, D. Van Nostrand Co., 1962.

Cope, Sir Zachary, *The Royal College of Surgeons of England: A History*. London, Anthony Bland, Ltd., 1959.

Crichton, M., *Five Patients, the Hospital Explained*. New York, Knopf, 1970.

Eckstein, Gustav, *The Body Has a Head*. New York, Harper & Row, 1970.

Fulton, J. F., *Harvey Cushing, A Biography*. Springfield, Thomas, 1946.

Garrison, F. H., *An Introduction to the History of Medicine*. Philadelphia, W. B. Saunders Co., 1929.

Meade, R., *An Introduction to the History of General Surgery*. Philadelphia, W. B. Saunders Co., 1968.

Netter, Frank H., *The Ciba Collection of Medical Illustrations, Heart, Volume 5*. Summit, CIBA, 1969.

Riesman, D., *The Story of Medicine in the Middle Ages*. New York, Hoeber, 1935.

Roueche, B., *Curiosities of Medicine*. Boston, Little, Brown, 1958.

Selzer, Arthur, *The Heart: Its Function in Health and Disease*. Berkeley, University of California Press, 1966.

Wilson, J. L., *Handbook of Surgery*. 4th ed. Los Altos, Lange Medical Publications, 1969.

Zimmerman, L. M. and Veith, I., *Great Ideas in the History of Surgery*. Baltimore, Williams and Wilkins Co., 1961.

ARTICLES

Barnard, C. N., "A Human Cardiac Transplant: An Interim Report of a Successful Operation Performed at Groote Schuur Hospital, Cape Town." *South African Medical Journal*, Vol. 41 (1967).

"Basic Research into why the Heart Fails." *Medical World News* (May 8, 1970).

Beall, Bricker, et al., "Surgical Management of Cardiovascular Trauma." *Medical Communications*, Department of Surgery, Baylor College of Medicine, Houston (1969).

Carrel, A., "Results of Transplantation of Blood Vessels, Organs and Limbs." *Journal of the American Medical Association*, Vol. 51 (1908).

"Cardiac Disease and Its Emotional Components." *Recent Developments in Psychiatry* (October, 1969).

"Cardiac Replacement." *Modern Medicine* (May 4, 1970), p. 1.

Castelnuovo-Tedesco, P., "How Cardiac Surgeons Look at Transplantation." *Seminars in Psychiatry* (January, 1971).

Cooley, Liotta, et al., "Orthotopic Cardiac Prosthesis for Two-Staged Cardiac Replacement." *The American Journal of Cardiology*, Vol. 24 (November, 1969).

Cope, Sir Zachary, "William Cheselden and the Separation of the Barbers from the Surgeons." *Annual of the Royal College of Surgery* (January, 1953).

DeBakey and Diethrich, "Acquired Diseases of the Aorta." *Current Therapy* (1969).

DeBakey, et al., "Atherosclerotic Occlusive Disease." *Medical Communications*, Baylor College of Medicine, Houston (1968).

DeBakey, et al., "Human Cardiac Transplantation: Clinical Experience." *The Journal of Thoracic and Cardiovascular Surgery*, Vol. 58, No. 3 (September, 1969).

DeBakey, Diethrich, et al., "Surgical Treatment of Coronary Heart Disease." *Department of Medical Illustration*, Baylor College of Medicine, Houston (1970).

DeBakey, Hall, et al., "Orthotropic Cardiac Prosthesis: Preliminary Experiments in Animals with Biventricular Artificial Heart." *Cardiovascular Research Center Bulletin* (April–June, 1969).

Diethrich, DeBakey, et al., "Preservation of the Human Heart." Baylor College of Medicine and the Cardiovascular Research and Training Center, Houston (1970).

Edson, L., "The Transplantation of the Species." *Esquire* (December, 1969).

Hardy, J. D., et al., "Heart Transplantation in Dogs, Procedures, Physiologic Problems and Results in 142 Experiments." *Surgery*, Vol. 60 (1966).

Hardy, J. D., et al., "Heart Transplantation in Man: Development Studies and Report of a Case." *Journal of the American Medical Association*, Col. 188 (1964).

Hazan, S. J., "Psychiatric Complications Following Cardiovascular Surgery." *The Journal of Thoracic and Cardiovascular Surgery*, Vol. 51, No. e, pp. 307–319.

Kennedy, Janet A., et al., "The Influence of Emotions on the Outcome of Cardiac Surgery: A Predictive Study." *Bulletin of The New York Academy of Medicine*, Vol. 42, No. 10 (1966).

Kraft, Irvin A., "Psychiatric Complications of Cardiac Transplantation." *Seminars in Psychiatry* (to be published).

Lazarus and Hagens, et al., "Prevention of Psychosis Following Open Heart Surgery." *The American Journal of Psychiatry*, Vol. 124, No. 9 (March, 1968).

Messmer, Nora, Leachman, Cooley, "Survival Times After Cardiac Allografts." *The Lancet*, London (May 10, 1969).

"A National Program to Conquer Heart Disease, Cancer and Stroke." *The President's Commission Report*, U.S. Government Printing Office (1964).

Nora, Cooley, et al., "Medical and Surgical Management of Anomalous Origin of the Left Coronary Artery from the Pulmonary Artery." *Pediatrics*, Vol. 42, No. 3 (September, 1968).

"People With Other People's Hearts." *Life* (January 10, 1969).

Quinn, J. and Bloom, M., "The Surgeons." *The New York Daily News*, 5-part series (September 8–12, 1969).

Reinhard, H., "Heart Transplant, The Whole World Watches." *Modern Hospital* (July, 1970).

Schwartz, et. al., "Basic Science and Cardiac Transplantation." *Cardiovascular Research Center Bulletin*, Houston (October, 1969).

Shearer, L., "Dr. Michael DeBakey." *Parade* (May 16, 1965).

Sprague, H. B., et al., "Examination of the Heart." Parts One, Two, Three, and Four. *American Heart Association* (1967).

"The Texas Tornado." *Time* (May 28, 1965).

"If Your Child Has a Congenital Heart Defect." *American Heart Association* (1967).